the Ultimate Guide
to Sex through
Pregnancy and
Motherhood

the Ultimate Guide to Sex through Pregnancy and Motherhood

Passionate, Practical Advice for Moms

by Madison Young

CLEiS
PRESS

Published in the United States by Cleis Press, an imprint of Start Midnight, LLC, 101 Hudson Street, Thirty-Seventh Floor, Suite 3705, Jersey City, NJ 07302.

Printed in the United States.
Cover design: Scott Idleman/Blink
Cover photograph: iStock Photos
Text design: Frank Wiedemann

First Edition.
10 9 8 7 6 5 4 3 2 1

Trade paper ISBN: 978-1-62778-152-7
E-book ISBN: 978-1-62778-161-9

I dedicate this book to a new generation of mothers, learning to love ourselves and to finding intimacy and pleasure in our every day. To a new generation of children, growing up with a knowledge and love of their bodies and selves along with the skills to navigate the giving and receiving of affection. May we all find profound pleasure and embrace the beauty and love that exists within all of us just as we are.

"Last night, I found a cheddar Goldfish in my vagina."

—Colin Nissan, *The New Yorker*

Contents

Preface

WELCOME TO *THE ULTIMATE* *Guide to Sex through Pregnancy and Motherhood!* I wrote this guide in hopes that it will be a written sanctuary for you—for all of us. A place where we can remember to breathe; a place where we can grow together—physically and emotionally. A retreat from the social expectations and unyielding heaps of advice that we receive as women, through pregnancy and then into motherhood. This is not a book that promises to give you all the answers. But it is a book that promises to support you in your own individual journey, through your own relationship to your body, your child, and your partner. It is a space that is free of judgment and that instead offers tools to guide you toward your own truth. It is a space where you will change, evolve, and transform. It is a space that you can return to time and time again to find different answers within yourself. You will discover new gems of wisdom, because you have changed; the same passages will bring about new emotions, new enlightenment in your body and mind, new creative sparks of inspiration in the bedroom, and new questions and answers for how you guide your children through their own relationship to their bodies, relationships, and sexuality. This book is a place you can return to, and within it you will find loving acceptance and support, along with the voices of many friends—sharing their experiences, their stories, their honest and candid lives as mothers. This is a place where our differences are celebrated and our shared humanity is cherished. You are entering a space in which we acknowledge that our bodies are not void of desire for intimacy and sizzling sex during pregnancy or motherhood. You are entering a safe space. One that is filled with love, and that was carefully constructed with great intent to support you in your journey. This book is a conversation. Feel free to talk back to its pages, write in the margins, pass it among other moms in your community, read it at night with your partner, or propose reading it in your local moms' group. Read it together. Talk about it. Add your own stories. Speak your story aloud. Your voice matters. You matter. You are love. You are pleasure. As you peel back the pages of this book, may pleasure, inspiration, and radical love fill your heart, body, and mind. May this book be a comforting embrace and tickle your heart with its inky words and earthy scent. Welcome.

Introduction and My Journey

WELCOME TO *THE ULTIMATE* *Guide to Sex through Pregnancy and Motherhood!* I wrote this book because I struggled to find the resources I needed during my pregnancy and postpartum to support my shifting identity and desires. It was an awkward learning experience full of trial and error, and as I reached out to other mothers around me, I found that they were struggling too. We became a resource for one another, forming the Sexy Mamas Social Club and along the way meeting sex-positive therapists, wellness providers, parenting and sex coaches, and medical practitioners. This book is a culmination of five years of hands-on research that I have gathered and shared through many of my mother-hood and sexuality workshops, as well as the many diverse voices of sexy mamas I've met in our community who are sharing their own personal journeys and experiences for the first time.

As a sex educator, erotic filmmaker, longtime sexual adventurer, and someone who has worked in the realm of sexuality for over a decade, I thought that I knew everything there was to know about what I liked and how I liked it. Pregnancy and motherhood shook all of what I thought I knew about myself and sent me flying deep down a surreal rabbit hole. Much like Alice as she somersaults into a new and strange world, I found myself contemplating the question "Who are you?" and, for the first time, struggling to answer.

Who was I? I was Madison Young, and I liked rough sex: tight bondage with hemp rope, accompanied by face slapping and nipple clamps...didn't I? I followed the white rabbit into a surreal landscape that became curiouser and curiouser, one that included an unfamiliar body that seemed to grow and shrink in the most bizarre ways until I truly no longer understood or recognized it.

You know the scene in *Alice in Wonderland* when Alice eats a bite of cake and grows to such an enormous size that her head and limbs break right out the roof and door and windows? Well, that's how I felt ballooning up sixty pounds during my pregnancy. My round, pregnant belly became so large that I couldn't see my precious vulva any longer! My breasts grew two cup sizes, from an A to a C—which, for someone who has never had cleavage, was a very strange experience—and postpartum, my nipples would squirt out milk when I sneezed or laughed. I felt out of control, and I wondered if I would ever know my body again.

As I wandered through my nine months of preggo Wonderland, this was just a fraction of my emotional landscape. There were wonderful, brilliant moments as well. Pregnancy challenged me and humbled me in the most amazing ways. It was like having a life coach that taught me the importance of being absolutely present and in the moment. This skill would prepare me for motherhood.

When we talk about sex and motherhood, we are talking about so much more than sexual techniques. We are talking about the emotional roller coaster that accompanies the huge transformations that pregnancy and motherhood bring—including hormonally. We are also talking about loving ourselves as we are in our bodies, in this moment—self-care, self-acceptance, and compassion for one's self. We are talking about identity, desire, communication, and relationship dynamics. We are talking about body politics, the importance of sleep, how breastfeeding affects sexual desire and body image, creative date nights for exhausted parents, and postpartum depression. We are talking about how to cultivate intimacy with a partner while experiencing sleep deprivation and how to explore new roles and sexual adventures with a partner in this new phase of life.

In this book, we will tackle all of these topics and guide you through this surreal landscape of experiencing pregnancy and motherhood as a sexual being. Because yes, mothers are still sexual beings, and just because we are now taking on the role of parents doesn't mean that we have to sacrifice intimacy, partner connection, pleasure, and orgasms. In fact, it's incredibly important as parents that we model healthy, loving relationships with our partners and a healthy relationship with our own bodies. This modeling sets a foundation for our children as they grow older—how they will share affection with others, the relationships they will develop, and the way they view their bodies. We will talk more about this, as well as how to set a healthy foundation for conversations around intimacy, consent, and shared affection, in Chapter 18.

In this guide you will find the tools you need to find your grounded path, find your pleasure, and relax into this otherworldly experience. Above all, know that you are not alone. Motherhood has the capability to crack our hearts open in a remarkable way, allowing us to feel love, connection, and pleasure on an entirely new level. So let's venture forward together, past the myths and fantasies of what we believe motherhood or pregnancy should be. Together, let's discover pleasure in who we are, as we are, and in pregnancy and motherhood as they are.

In this book I will share with you my findings as a sex educator and sex coach to parents, as well as my personal experiences throughout pregnancy and motherhood. I've also brought in the voices of many other mothers and experts on parenting, wellness, and sexuality to give us their points of view and add their voices to the book. It's important as we journey on to remember that no one person experiences sexuality, sexual desire, pregnancy, or motherhood in exactly the same way. Experiences will vary, which is why I have tried to bring in a variety of voices and perspectives for this book. The way that you experience desire on your own time is perfectly okay. Loving and accepting ourselves as we are and releasing expectations from others is truly the first step to experiencing profound sexual pleasure.

My Journey Down the Rabbit Hole

My journey toward motherhood was a humbling one. Among other things, it taught me that we are more than we know we are and that everything evolves and transforms with each and every breath. It continues to teach me that life is never as you expect it to be. Motherhood, as well, is not as I expected it to be.

When I was pregnant, I researched all the different models of parenting. I thought about what kind of parent I might be. What style of parenting would best fit me and my politics and my way of life? I was able to make what seemed at the time like concrete decisions: I wanted a natural childbirth, I would use only cloth diapers, I would co-sleep and breastfeed my child, and I would be back to work two weeks postpartum (did I even really need that much time?). But the reality of parenthood and pregnancy hit me hard well before I ever met my child.

After I discovered I was pregnant, I had to examine how motherhood would affect my career, my body, and my life, and whether those were changes that I wanted. After some brief meditation, I decided that yes, I wholeheartedly wanted to journey into motherhood.

I was on tour for the majority of my pregnancy, traveling to different cities, countries, and continents and taking advantage of early boarding privileges for pregnant ladies. Score! I had a relatively easy pregnancy, but my partner wasn't around until the third trimester, and negotiating my way through all the emotional and hormonal roller coasters of pregnancy was tough.

Then there were the body image issues. I love my body, but I did not expect to gain as much weight as I did. I'm five foot two and usually weigh in between 117 and 124 pounds; by the time I was in labor, I was tipping the scales at 180. My mother had gained fifty pounds with each of her two pregnancies, and I thought to myself, *That won't be me.* I walk a minimum of five miles a day just commuting, I exercise, and I'm vegan. There was no way I'd gain as much as my mother. But...I did. And my line of work didn't allow me to hide under large maternity garments.

As both a body-based performance artist and adult performer, I was often naked. I vividly remember my last trip to LA before the birth of my child. I was performing in a MILF film—the first MILF film in which I was going to be the MILF. I was playing an expectant mother interviewing babysitters for her child-to-be. During the interview, I end up seducing the sitter. I was over 170 pounds, thirty years old and thirty-seven weeks pregnant, paired up with a one hundred-pound, nineteen-year-old girl. At thirty-seven weeks, I couldn't even see my vulva anymore!

Before the film shoot, I took a luxurious shower. For the first time in well over a decade, I found myself nervous about a shoot. In front of the camera was where I felt at home, but at thirty-seven weeks pregnant, I didn't recognize my body anymore. I dried off and stared at my naked body in the mirror, large and round. My butt, for the first time in my life, looked flat in the mirror in comparison to the roundness of my belly and my swollen legs and ankles beneath me.

I closed my eyes and felt my breasts, shifting my hips back and forth, swaying and breathing, generating erotic energy in my vessel. I looked up, smiled, and said, "You are beautiful. You are sexy. Your body is a powerful container for erotic energy. You are a conduit for delicious pleasure." I kept repeating these words, seducing myself, staring into the mirror, touching my breasts and my round belly, finding my cunt below and all its juiciness. My physical container (my body) had expanded, and so my energy and pleasure within, my love for myself and for others, needed to expand and grow too.

Despite the body-image challenges that arose during pregnancy, my sexual appetite was robust—though erratic! Although I felt challenged and terrified by my body changing noticeably every week, every month, I also felt radically turned on by it and empowered by my growing body and my curves, by having cleavage for the first time in my life and experiencing an element of the sexual goddess.

I also know that my experience is not the experience of every woman—that just as our desires and bodies are all unique, sexual snowflakes prior to pregnancy, that each pregnancy and the sexual desires that accompany that pregnancy also vary widely. We are all unique individuals, and there is no need to tie yourself down with expectations of how you should feel.

Being a sexy mama doesn't mean always feeling sexy; sometimes you may also feel sadness or a lack of desire. It might mean caring for yourself as an individual, or just wanting to connect with your partner by holding hands. Intimacy may look like your partner rubbing your feet and legs as you eat your favorite ice cream.

Self-care is sexy, and it's a key element of nurturing your sexuality. Learning to honor your desires and needs is one of the first steps to developing a healthy relationship with your sexual self. This experience of nurturing yourself will be further challenged when your child arrives. When you have a small child who needs to be nurtured on a full-time basis, it's easy for your needs and desires—including showers and eating!—to take a backseat. No wonder so many moms face challenges in finding their way back to their sexual identity—if we can't meet our basic needs of sleep, food, and hygiene, how do we intend to find, experience, and share pleasure with ourselves or our partners?

If there is a single seed of wisdom that you take from this guide, I hope that it is this: Breathe deeply, inhale your reality, and exhale compassion. Be gentle with yourself. Create time for yourself—even five minutes a day—because nourishment is essential. You are beautiful and radiant just as you are, and you deserve pleasure and connection—don't allow the world to shame or guilt you into thinking that you don't. We may have entered Wonderland, but that doesn't mean we have to scamper and struggle back up the rabbit hole. Stay for a while. Accept the surreal as your reality of the moment rather than struggling against it.

A SEXY MAMA'S POV
WITH AYA DE LEON

In college, shortly after I stopped using the Pill, I discovered fluid leaking from my breasts. I called the university health services and they were utterly clueless, except to assure me that if it was happening on both sides, it couldn't be cancer. Over the next two decades, it became clear that I had a hormonal imbalance, and eventually I stopped having my period because my body thought it was already pregnant.

In my thirties, I began to have discomfort in my vagina during sex. At first, I thought it was as a result of the hormonal imbalance. I later learned that it was unrelated. Of course, these two things are connected because they both take place in my body, but one does not cause the other. Eventually, the vaginal pain was diagnosed as vulvodynia. This is a sort of catchall, garbage-can term for pain in the vulva or vagina. It's the equivalent of referring to both a migraine and blunt force trauma to the skull as a "pain in the head." But of course, when it comes to women's genitals and sexuality, the medical industry is notoriously clueless and insensitive.

In fact, vulvodynia came to the attention of medical researchers in the 1800s, but then Sigmund Freud explained this and various other women's sexual health concerns with another garbage-can term, "frigidity," and there was no more research done for one hundred years. So when my doctor referred me to a GYN specialist, he poked around a bit and gave me a prescription for a topical anesthetic. Yes, people, he told me that the answer to pain during sex was to numb my vagina. I thought, Are you kidding me? I'm trying to have pleasure here, not just close my eyes and think of the Empire. I didn't use the prescription for months. But then, finally, I was sick of the discomfort and I broke down and used it. Imagine my despair when I slathered on tons of it and it didn't work. Somehow, I was experiencing numbness and pain at the same time.

I was really demoralized about getting any help. My sex life with my partner suffered a great deal, mostly due to the hopelessness. Eventually, I saw a pelvic physical therapist, who explained that the pain was actually muscular, but I felt it on the surface of the skin. She had me do Kegels and use dilators, and voilà! Problem solved.

A few years later, my (male) partner and I decided we wanted to have a baby. So I needed to use the dilators, and I also needed to take medicine for the hormonal imbalance to make me fertile. Sex with an agenda of getting pregnant was so foreign, because I had spent so many years trying not to get pregnant. But it happened immediately after the endocrinologist got me on the right dose. And also immediate was the rise in my sex drive during pregnancy. My partner was startled by how much I was interested in sex all the time—that is, all the time when I wasn't worried about all the usual concerns that first-time moms have. I was also worried about the vulvodynia. Would my vaginal muscles clench when I was giving birth? Would it be really painful? I asked my midwife, and she couldn't find a clear answer. As it turned out, I had a lovely home birth in a tub, which pretty much cured my vulvodynia for good. Stretching to accommodate a baby seems to have defeated that chronic clenching of my vaginal muscles.

Since we became parents, however, the new challenge is finding time and energy to have sex. As a wage-earning mom who is always working on various writing projects, I find the bed most seductive for sleeping. But as my partner and I dig out from under the biggest challenges of new parenthood, we have a newfound appreciation for each other. We treasure the stolen moments when we can enjoy our bodies beyond being laps to sit on, horsies to ride, arms to lift someone sleepy, and machines to do all the earning and domestic work of a family. These moments are lovely, hard earned, and precious.

Discovering Your New Sexuality

I HAD SO MANY ideas about how my labor would go down. I wanted to labor at home as much as possible. I wanted it to be as natural as possible, with no epidural and little to no medical intervention. I knew I was capable of birthing a child. I was capable of anything...but I wasn't expecting a forty-seven-hour labor!

Around forty hours in, I accepted the offer of an epidural after receiving the news that my cervix was swollen and my blood pressure (and baby's blood pressure) was rising. I felt partially defeated, but continued on— what choice did I have? I realized this baby had ideas of its own and was coming into this world the way that it wanted to, on its own terms.

Then there was the baby. This baby. This baby was there and screaming and did it ever stop screaming? No matter the number of Beatles songs that I quietly sang to my child or the number of tie-dyed onesies I bought, this kid was not going to give peace a chance. My kid was a rebel with a cause, a scream-core anarchist from the start.

I deeply loved my spirited child. I loved our sleepless nights together. The intimacy of nursing and rocking late into the night. The deep, sweeping vortex of new motherhood that made the rest of the world nothing but a blur with a singular focus of nurturing this tiny creature.

I had fallen deeply in love with the new dominant persona in the house, my child, and I was experiencing an all-new type of service and devotion as I saw my whole world reflected in the eyes of this new part of our family. A new relationship to nurture. Another person with needs and desires, and an individual in the making. Despite the intimacy and bond I felt for our colicky child, I desperately craved more intimacy with my partner.

Our doctor had advised us to wait until after my six-week checkup before penetrative sex, which felt like a long wait! But I love non-penetrative play so much that it didn't hinder our intimacy during that time. I adore performing oral sex, cocks and cunts alike. I love to have something in my mouth to seduce with my tongue, my lips, and my throat. During that six-week waiting period we enjoyed a great deal of blow jobs, analingus, and oral stimulation of my breasts. (Check out Chapter 20 for my favorite oral sex techniques.) And there were other aspects of live-out-loud sexuality that sidestepped penetration, like the creative sexual world of kink! (Which you can read more about in Chapter 21.)

But there were other things that just didn't work as well or as easily.

Things That Go Squirt...and Things That Don't

As someone who has often experienced ejaculation when engaging in G-spot stimulation, I was not a novice when it came to squirting. However, milk squirting from my breasts—that was something new. Especially within the first few weeks postpartum, my breasts were incredibly engorged with milk, and if I sneezed, laughed, or became aroused, I would be leaking and squirting milk from my nipples. I felt like a teenage boy coming in his pants at the first glimpse of something that he found arousing, but I was coming from my breasts! This was both fascinating and, honestly, a little embarrassing. I'm usually very comfortable with bodily fluids, but this was a new bodily fluid, and something that I felt I had little control over. It didn't last forever; my milk supply chilled out after a few weeks and I only occasionally experienced premature lactation after that, but it is something that I will never forget.

As I mentioned, ejaculation was no foreign concept to me. It was a sexual experience that I quite enjoyed and that I continued to experience throughout my pregnancy. But after I birthed my child, my well ran dry.

I stopped ejaculating. I was terrified by this. Why was this happening? Would I never ejaculate again? Had I traded in my wet orgasms for motherhood? I was panicky about a lot of the postpartum experience. I saw a distinct line in the sand. On one side lay life before motherhood; on the other, motherhood, with its challenges and uncertainties. But like everything, life continues to evolve and move and shift and change.

Our bodies respond to stress. Stressors like lack of sleep and the anxiety of caring for a new child—as well as any tensions we might be experiencing with a partner or at work or around loss of identity—can affect our arousal response cycle, our sexual experiences, and our reactions to stimulation, such as ejaculation. Also, post–vaginal birth, the PC (pubococcygeus) muscles are stretched and weakened. These are the same muscles used to release and push ejaculate forth out of the body.

Kegels can help in strengthening these muscles again, but it takes time to rebuild muscle strength. Along with weakened PC muscles, new motherhood caused such physical and emotional stress to my body that I wasn't able to ejaculate for a little more than a year. I did experience plenty of hot sex and incredible orgasms, and when my body was ready, I started to ejaculate again.

Other moms I have spoken with have told me that they didn't start to ejaculate until after giving birth. That birth was this orgasmic experience that opened up the gateway to releasing this entirely new level of pleasure for them. Each experience is valid and different, and will vary based on our bodies, relationships, and emotional experiences around birth and postpartum life.

The important thing is to know that our bodies are really smart, and that we can't push them to do something that they don't want to do. Listen to your body. Listen to what it needs, and let it respond to sexual stimuli in its own time in a way that makes sense to it in that moment. Be patient and present in the moment, and honor your body in its present experience.

It's common to attempt to try everything that you enjoyed before or during pregnancy, and to expect the same arousal experience and reaction. It's what we know. But letting go of the past and connecting with what your body desires right now is a key element to building a road map to your new sexual identity as a mother. Your maps and destinations will continue to change and evolve throughout your life. So let go of the past, don't worry about the future, and create a road map for the now.

The Road Map to a Sexy Mama

Let's locate where you are right now and map out possible destinations to include in your travels as a sexy mama. This exercise will assist you in discovering where you are right now and create inspiration and confidence for what you might want to explore. Remember, it's about the journey, not the destination.

Reading your Compass and Identifying Home Base

Before we venture into other lands, it's important to establish where we are starting from. An excellent way to identify your home base is to do daily check-ins with yourself. It's important to allow space to release your thoughts and feelings and create a place for reflection. A written or video journal can be a radically cathartic emotional release and provide space for your voice to be heard—by you. This is important, for we must first hear our own voices and needs before we can articulate our needs and desires to others.

I really enjoyed using a video journal or even an audio journal, since for the first few months of motherhood I felt so brain-dead that writing a complete sentence was an utter challenge. Collecting my thoughts and ramblings on a video or audio recording was easier for me. I generally used a program like Photo Booth on my laptop, or the voice memo or video camera function on my smartphone. If you are more of a visual person, you might want to try sketching in a sketchbook. This doesn't have to be polished; it's for your own eyes and your own reflection. It helps if you can use the same check-in questions each day. It doesn't have to be time consuming, and this should not take away from self-care. Even a timed five minutes of this practice can be radically helpful.

Here are a few check-in prompts you may want to consider using:

- What is one way that I engaged in self-care today?
- Today I'm sending love and radiant energy to _____ (name a part of your body) because _____.
- Today I felt an intimate connection to _____ (name a person or thing) by or through _____ (name the act that served as the conduit for that connection).
- Today I felt gratitude for _____. I'll express my gratitude by _____.
- Today I felt a desire for more _____ in my life. I will let more _____ into my life by _____.
- One thing I love about my partner (or self) today is _____.
- One thing I love about my body today is _____.
- One way in which my partner could nourish my heart and body today is _____. (Share this with your partner.)
- One way in which I'd like to connect intimately with my partner today is _____.
- The part of my body that is most in need of touch, connection, warmth, and love right now is _____.
- The type of touch I'm craving right now is _____.
- One new thing I want to try is _____.
- One obstacle I faced today was _____. When I was met with this obstacle, I felt _____. When faced with obstacles like this, I'll show myself love and compassion by _____.

As you can see, these questions hold space for your self-reflection and honor your desires and needs on each day. The type of touch or connection that you need one day might not be what you need the next day. These check-ins will give you the emotional GPS coordinates for where you are and where you might be interested in exploring on any given day. Try to make it part of your daily practice. I always like to do mine during a soak in the bathtub, but you could do yours while your little one is napping, or while you're strolling with your child or taking your child for a walk in the carrier. When you are able to identify your needs, it becomes much easier to articulate your needs and desires to your partner.

You might find that occasionally your eyes are bigger than your stomach. Be gentle with yourself. I'm going to say this throughout the book, because it's perhaps the most difficult thing to do as a mom. It's important for us to identify our cravings and our needs and our desires and then do what we can. We won't always be able to meet all of our desires or all of the desires of our partner or child. And that is okay. Small steps can create radical change and a huge difference. Keep with it. Before having a child, maybe self-care looked like soaking in a hot tub with your girlfriends or going for a spa day. But in the first few months of motherhood, self-care might look like having a coffee around the corner by yourself while you read a book for thirty minutes, or having an evening bubble bath while your partner rocks the baby, or asking a friend to hold your child or take your child for a stroll while you eat a meal, or buying your favorite lotion and taking the time to apply it after a shower, or going in for waxing! Maybe, instead of a mani/pedi, you only have time for a mani while the baby is sleeping. You will discover your little nibbles of self-care, and they will still be effective and nourishing to your spirit and body. Slowly, you will hit a new stride in your self-care and sexual well-being as you reclaim your sexuality and your daily desires and discover your new sexual identity as a mother.

A SEXY MAMA'S POV
WITH HARMONY NILES

My baby started losing weight at around five weeks old. She was so small, so thin. It was breaking my heart to look at her, and I didn't know what the problem was.

I wasn't producing enough milk to support her growth. I'm slowly starving her, I thought. I know that sounds harsh, but that's exactly how I felt. I was devastated and full of self-blame. I wasn't able to be a good mother.

Tests were not able to find anything wrong with me. I started a punishing regimen of pumping five times a day. Since I was doing childcare by myself, I was exhausted all of the time. I was on an expensive and difficult-to-get drug called domperidone, plus enough fenugreek to make me smell like an IHOP. My milk production had some improvement, but not enough.

It later became clear through working with a craniosacral therapist that my daughter had a dropped palate. She was unable to draw the nipple into her mouth very far, because it would choke her, so her sucking was very shallow. That set my milk production to be very low. My breasts were never emptied, which would have triggered greater production.

Feeling like an absolute failure, I started to make her a homemade baby formula with a recipe that I had gotten from the Weston A. Price Foundation nutrition website. By the time she was six months old, I was thoroughly exhausted and demoralized, and she was much more interested in an easy-to-drink bottle than in my difficult breasts.

My boyfriend adored breasts—breasts of all kinds,

and especially milky breasts. I had been feeling too tense, my milk too scarce, to allow ourselves to have fun with that. But now I thought, what the hell! He nursed from my breasts as part of our lovemaking. The next morning I had the experience which they say happens three to five days after the birth of your child. I woke up to find the bed wet with milk and my breasts engorged. I cried.

I shared this story with a lactation consultant, and she said, "Oh, yeah, that can really help a lot." I was so mad that she hadn't told me this before! I had been willing to do anything! Why wouldn't she suggest the easy, cheap, and pleasurable way? Pure prudishness.

Getting in Touch with Your Sexual Self

MY POSTPARTUM BODY BROUGHT up painful, deeply ingrained memories of the transitions and awkwardness that accompanied puberty. I was used to feeling confident, empowered, and present in my body. Now I felt weak, confused, and detached from whatever alien flesh-bag my spirit was housed in. Where did this mutant body come from? Why did this feel like a huge, cruel joke, that I was now supposed to care for my child in a body that I didn't know, recognize, or want to be in? I didn't know how to move around in this body. My joints were soft and gummy and not ready for high heels. My breasts were laughable—one was an entire cup size bigger than the other due to my child developing a strong preference for the left one. Thanks for that!

When I sneezed or laughed, my engorged breasts squirted out milk, like one of those flowers on a clown's lapel that squirt water—just like that, but with milk and it was not funny. It didn't feel funny; it felt like the joke was on me, over and over again. And I could not complete a sentence. I'm an articulate woman who generally can't stop talking when I'm asked about something like sexuality or feminism, and yet, as I stepped across the threshold of motherhood, I found myself without words, crying when my child was crying, crying when my child was laughing. Crying and covered in bodily fluids and mumbling incoherent, fragmented thoughts—incomplete words, sounds. Perhaps, like my newborn, I was learning to speak again.

There is a loss of identity that comes with motherhood. A feeling that you are waiting for something, for time to pass, for a sign that you're not failing. It seems clear that this is some sort of transitional period, and yet there is no clear defining marker of how long it will last, how long you will feel this way. Perhaps the most frightening thought is this: *What in the world could I be transitioning into? What does that look like? What will that be like?*

So instead we reside in this middle ground. This state of change. Neither the Hulk nor Bruce Banner. A tadpole with legs, a Transformer that is not quite sure what it will transform into for the first time. And yet in the midst of all this transition and awkwardness and squirting of milk and feelings of depression and inadequacy, perhaps more than ever, I craved acceptance and intimacy. But what do our sexual identities look like when we are in the middle of an identity crisis as new moms?

Well, our sexual identities might look a little fragmented, and that's okay. I believe that intense transitions (like becoming a mother for the first time) are this experience in which who we were bursts into thousands of tiny pieces, and those little pieces of ourselves get swirled around like glitter in a snow globe. All of us is there, just fragmented and swirling around in this watery base of emotions, and we're never quite sure where the pieces are going to land.

One of the things that helped me to gain some control was to locate and state my emotions, and then let them go. I remember several scenarios where my newborn baby had a massive blowout and I found myself covered in poop. Once I was actually giving a talk at UC Berkeley while nursing my child in a sling, and my child had a huge blowout in the midst of my talk. I was covered in poop in front of a classroom full of students. I remember many other moments, such as at gallery art exhibits, when my wee one spit up on me. During these experiences, I'd acknowledge, "I am covered in poop. This sucks." Then I'd clean up and let it go.

Perhaps one of the most beautiful and helpful visualization tools that I used was to picture myself as a reed and tell myself that the emotion I was experiencing was not me. I was not the emotion; I was the vessel, and through my breath I could move sensations and emotions through my body. I had the power to release them. If I was experiencing a feeling of shame or awkwardness in the locker room of the gym while I was changing, that was okay. I could acknowledge that feeling of shame and awkwardness about my breasts being lopsided and my belly big and tiger-striped. I would stop right there in front of my locker rather than rushing to cover myself up, and release the feeling with a big exhale, acknowledging and releasing shame and making room for a new emotion. And I would smile. It felt so good to release those negative feelings and make room for new positive feelings about my "now" body instead of focusing on my pre-mommy body or my future body.

Regaining strength, power, and control over your body, and experiencing radical acceptance of your body the way it is, are all building blocks toward reclaiming your body and loving yourself during this transformation. Here is a list of sexy mama tools to add to your toolbox. These tools will aid you in your journey toward embracing your sexual desire, body, and identity as a mother.

Do something for your body that feels good physically—Dance! Turn on some of your favorite music and jam out! Find excuses to move your body, whether it's walking with your baby, dancing, or doing yoga. Find a way to move your body that feels good to you now. Moving your body helps to increase blood flow, adrenaline, and endorphins. It will also help you in finding your path back to your body. Something as simple as hip circles can start to bring erotic, loving energy back into your body. So get moving. Move with your baby, move on your own, move with your partner, and let out a wild call into the world that tethers you to the unified ecstasy of all humankind.

Homework: Create a playlist of songs that make you feel amazing and inspired and make you want to move your body! Music is a wonderful motivator for movement—try a get-up-and-dance playlist, a sexy playlist for intimate time with your partner, and slow-dancing music for dancing and swaying your little one to sleep.

Go to the mirror and look at yourself—Try it, right now. Take a long look and release whatever comes up emotionally. Use your breath and exhale any sadness, any fear, and any anxieties. Allow those emotions to flow out of your vessel. Release them. Now, settle into a place of acceptance and bliss, in the perfection of existing in this very moment. In the beauty of standing here in the midst of this journey. Recognize the curves of your body, the strength and determination in your eyes, the fullness of your breasts, the bow of your lips. Find a part of your body that turns you on. A part of you that your eyes gravitate toward and that you recognize as full of life and beauty.

Wear something that turns you on in your sexy mama body—The clothes that used to look super sexy on us in our pre-mama life or even during pregnancy are not likely to be the clothes that look super sexy on us post-partum or during early motherhood. Find clothes that look sexy and feel sexy to you in your new sexy mama life. There is no one definition of what "sexy " looks like. In fact, what looks sexy on you will be the clothes that *feel* sexy on you. What textures feel really great on your skin right now? What textures or styles make you feel inspired and nourished and confi-dent? Those will be your sexy clothes. That might mean a killer pair of cowboy boots that totally turns you on. It might mean some silky under-wear that feels really smooth and luxurious against your skin right now.

The first Mother's Day that I celebrated as a mother, my daughter was two months old and my partner bought me this super-sexy pair of high-heeled Doc Martens. I needed stable, strong footwear to hike up and down the hills of San Francisco with my baby, but my femme side was dying to get back into a pair of heels. Badass mama black heeled boots allowed me to listen to what my body and my libido needed while making me feel sexy and confident in my expression of self.

I nursed my little one until she weaned from nursing at about eighteen months. So my tops and dresses required easy boob access. Button-down shirts, stretchy or silky camisoles, and a handful of nursing bras that didn't feel totally utilitarian and sterile were key to finding a balance between nourishing my sexual self and still caring for my infant. There are now more and more lingerie lines that are coming out with nursing and mater-nity lingerie! Check out Hot Milk and Dita Von Teese's nursing bras. For me, silky slips from vintage stores, silky robes, and sexy undies were all also a part of my new sexy mama wardrobe. A hot garter, waist cincher, vintage girdles, and luxurious stockings gave this sexy mama a new look as I made my way into motherhood. Something to keep in mind: You are in transition, and these things won't necessarily fit you in four months. So you might just want to keep that in mind when making purchases. But a handful of sexy wardrobe staples—items that really connect you back to your body, sensuality, and confidence—can be wondrous in your journey to finding your sexy mama identity.

Engage in touch and relax into it—Whether this means a mani/pedi or a massage or even the daily application of body lotion or a long luxurious shower or bath, start to move energy around in your body through receiving intimate touch and being present and accepting to the sensation and energy you're receiving.

When we are receiving touch, it's not a passive act. Slow down and become mindful of the sensation you are experiencing. Don't just rush past the experience of applying lotion to your legs, arms, and breasts, but really sink into the sensation and indulge in the moment. How do you feel in your body? Lean into that feeling, move it around in your body through touch, and start to really use your breath and intention to bring a consciousness to the sensuality of touch and sensation.

Practice affirmations, meditation, and yoga—We will talk more about these mindfulness tools in Chapter 8. Affirmations, meditation, and yoga can be powerful tools in our journey to a sexy mama life. Even if you are able to carve out just five minutes for meditation each day—time in which you are able to sit and let go of your thoughts, insecurities, expectations, and emotions and just acknowledge them and set them free, focusing on your inhale and exhale—you will notice a radical difference in your overall wellness, clarity, and ability to communicate with your partner and to communicate your sexual desires and needs.

Get in touch with nature—Become a sensualist and *slooooow down*. Our world praises being fast and moving quickly. As a result, we often rush past each moment in a hurry to get to the next. Try slowing down. By doing so, I've been able to experience each moment in life much more fully, and it has been helpful in my ability to release outside expectations and connect more deeply to my friends, the earth, my child, and my partner. My work doesn't suffer, but actually thrives creatively.

Slow down and experience the scent of the leaves as they fall in autumn, the touch of wind as it blows against your body and face, the tiny creatures like poky snails that come out after the rainfall. Listen to the birds, watch the careful work of bees as they gather pollen, stop and smell the flowers (literally), gaze at the stars and the moon.

You might be wondering what this has to do with your sexual self. When we relax and open ourselves to embracing and cultivating our sensual nature, we relax and open ourselves to experiencing pleasure with our connection to the world around us as well as with our partners.

Have your photo taken or take your own photos...naked—There are many female boudoir photographers and artists who focus on photography of women during pregnancy and postpartum. This can be a really empowering experience and a great way of really recognizing the beauty and sexuality that exists in you at this very moment. Not quite ready to step in front of a stranger's lens? Ask your partner to take photos of you, or take a series of postpartum self-portraits that capture your sexy mama identity. You can manifest these images either with a camera, timer, and tripod, or selfie-style with your smartphone.

Masturbate—As far as I'm concerned, there is no better way of getting your sexy mama groove back than exploring your sexual self on your own before reconnecting with partnered sex. When you give yourself the time and space to explore your own body and sexual desires, you are able to discover what works for you in your sexual self right now.

Masturbating now that you are a mom might look a little different. We find different pockets of time for self-love and touch. I find that making time in the shower or bath for masturbation works well for me. There are even waterproof toys—vibrating rubber duckies! And the showerhead can add a little pleasure to the sexy mama's sex life. I also love my incognito Crave vibrator necklace. I wear it everywhere I go! It looks just like a classy, beautiful pendant, and it charges through a USB plug in my computer. It's super sexy, and there is something I just love about always having my vibe with me no matter where I am.

Stop the negative talk—from both yourself and others—If you catch yourself engaging in negative self-talk, counter it with an affirmation. One example of negative self-talk that often found its way into my consciousness goes something like this: "I'm so squishy. I'm never going to be able to fit into my old clothes. I feel like a feeding sack for my baby. I want my body back!" It's totally natural to feel this way. And it's okay to give yourself time and space to mourn your previous life. But don't let it take control of your self-talk.

Try countering the negative self-talk with affirmations and positive self-talk. That's right—I'm encouraging you to have conversations with yourself! Either out loud, in your head, or on paper. The positive self-talk you use to counter that negative self-talk might look like this: "I know you're feeling out of place in your body. That can feel scary, and experiencing a body that is new and different can be difficult. This is difficult, but it won't last forever. This will change. You are beautiful and deserving of love exactly as you are in this moment."

Also, if you find your mind getting bogged down with negative self-talk, take five minutes and just purge all of those negative thoughts onto paper. Get them all out there, and then light a candle and burn it—burn all those negative thoughts and just release them. Let them go. Your light, beauty, and positive energy are so much stronger than those thoughts. Let them go. You don't need them anymore, and they are taking up room in your vessel that you need for love, compassion, and erotic energy.

USEFUL TOOLS IN THE TRANSITION FROM PREGNANCY TO MOTHERHOOD
WITH NATASHIA FUKSMAN, MA

Our bodies undergo major transitions during pregnancy and postpartum. I often correlate it with puberty—after you've gone through that process, you're never going to have your old body anymore. There isn't much conversation about the grief that occurs, or about ending a chapter of your life.

The tools that I've witnessed to have been of service during this transition are things like group support. It can be a non-facilitated group, but getting together regularly with women who are in or around the same transition period and learning how to have candid conversations about what you're experiencing can be immensely helpful.

For instance, in the six-session groups that I lead, we meet twice a week: once as a facilitated group, and the second time as a non-facilitated meetup. This gives a bit of guidance for women to have open and candid conversations with one another in a society that's so drenched in judgment towards women, towards mothers, towards parents, and about sex and bodies.

The facilitated portion really helps to set a tone for processing each one of our own judgments, and to let the women openly speak to one another. This process continues in the meetings those women have on their own. And often the women will continue to meet up after the group sessions are done.

INTERVIEW WITH MOOREA MALATT
PARENTING COACH, LACTATION EXPERT, AND THE FOUNDER OF SAVVY PARENTING

I had the great pleasure of interviewing Moorea Malatt, parenting coach and lactation expert, on many of the common concerns that arise for women regarding sex, bodies, and breastfeeding.

Madison: *I've had several moms quietly admit to me after discovering that I was a sex educator that they felt aroused or experienced sensations similar to orgasm during breastfeeding. From the conversations I've had, it seems there is a lot of shame packed into this topic, and I was wondering if you might be willing to unpack some of that for us and share with the readers some of the physiology around these feelings and this physical reaction.*

Moorea: *I have heard this same shame and worry from so many women. The cure for shame here is information about anatomical functions, sex, and breastfeeding. One of the first things we do to help the womb and vagina heal after birth is to put the baby on the breast. Breastfeeding causes the uterus to contract and even the vaginal muscles to tighten in very much the same way that for many of us breast play during sex lubes us up and makes us excited. Breastfeeding causes blood flow to the vagina and vulva. I find it both impossible and ludicrous to try to separate our sexual and maternal functions. Sex and motherhood are bosom buddies. Why would the birth of a child suddenly sever that breast-genital connection?*

Another cure for this shame about sexual feelings while breastfeeding may be to dive back into getting in touch—literally—with our mama bodies a bit sooner than we are told.

We are expected to be disconnected from our sexuality as soon as the baby is born and then for at least the first six weeks. By "sex," your midwife or MD likely means "intercourse," which could cause infection or pain. However, after a vaginal birth, clitoral stimulation and breast stimulation are both safe as soon as it is comfortable, and I believe it is important for moms to explore themselves sexually as mothers to help integrate those Madonna/whore parts of oneself that the patriarchy would like to force us to separate. I also hear so many moms express shame that they are randy before the six weeks are up. This is something to be celebrated. Listen to your body. I have heard women say that they sometimes need to masturbate after breastfeeding. This is not pedophilia. Your child is not turning you on. You are simply having a physiological chain reaction because you own a dual-function body part.

These sexual feelings and shame during breastfeeding usually first come up in those first postpartum weeks when we are getting to know our new body functions. These feelings usually pass, as breastfeeding becomes more of a mundane twelve-times-per-day part of life. Nipples also toughen up a bit, and women find they are less sensitive during breastfeeding if they just push through the challenge of those first few weeks.

Madison: How does breastfeeding affect a woman's sex life or sexual desire?

Moorea: I think women who were previously more into breast play before having a baby are the ones most changed by breastfeeding's effects on sex. Getting used *to a postpartum body in general can lessen desire, as can pure exhaustion.*

Breastfeeding can make women feel "touched out" and therefore not want to be physically intimate at the end of the day. Simply enjoying a movie next to one another or having an adult conversation can be intimate when mom simply cannot.

Madison: *How does breastfeeding affect a woman's body image?*

Moorea: *Pregnancy changes breasts, and then breastfeeding changes breasts some more. I am quite a "lactivist," but the articles that tell you breastfeeding will not change your breasts are setting you up for misery rather than preparing you to learn to love a changing body. Pregnancy and breastfeeding can change body image quite dramatically because they happen so fast compared to, say, the gradual changes of becoming older. Some women suddenly see themselves as sexier and more voluptuous because of the increase in breast volume and perkiness. Other women simply feel uncomfortable because they feel different from their usual self. Once the engorgement of the first few months subsides, some women notice that their breasts look larger but flatter or saggier because the skin has stretched somewhat, and it can be hard to come to terms with this change if it does not fit in with society's vision of the perfect breast. I had this challenge and felt that it was very cathartic to write funny poetry and draw pictures of my changing breasts, as well as to see many images of breastfeeding and mothers' breasts on social media.*

It isn't easy to suddenly love a whole new body. Anything you can do to feel sexy overall is helpful. I personally found sexier nursing bras to be helpful. And I think it is good to make a point to spend time alone with your breasts, noticing them and appreciating their purpose and then coming into sharing them with your partner from a place of self-appreciation.

Madison: *I've heard varying opinions from partners of moms—some partners are turned on by their partner lactating while others are weirded out by it, by the idea that a part of her body is pulling double duty as both a source of nourishment and an erogenous zone during sexual play. I've also heard from women who are lactating that they feel confused or not sexually confident with their breasts when they are breastfeeding, now that their breasts are a food source. What tips or advice do you have for lactating moms and their partners about coming to terms with their feelings around lactation and sexual play with breasts?*

Moorea: *As challenging as it is for some women to make the switch between being food source and sexy mutha, I also hear that women are challenged because they worry their partner will find the capacity for lactation (or breast leaking or even the new size!) to be strange or not sexy. The secret is that most people who enjoy having sex with female bodies (I would venture ninety percent of them) also enjoy the idea of pregnancy and lactation. The Internet has pregnancy and lactation porn sites for a reason. It is also extremely common for partners to try breast milk and like it! This sort of breast play is safe with a partner you are already fluid-bonded with.*

Start easy and slow, getting to know the breasts again together, and pay close attention to consent and timing. If breasts are full and baby is about to wake up to nurse, it may not be the most comfortable time for breast play physiologically or psychologically. Talk about it beforehand. "Do we stop or keep going if I'm leaking milk all over?"

I would be remiss to forget the partners that are turned off by lactation. It happens. I have spoken to at least fifteen male and female partners of clients or friends who have felt like this, and all have said that they wish they were into it but just are not. In this case I think we may be able to attempt to think of it less like a personal rejection and more like anal sex. Some people just can't go there. You are free to go there yourself. It is okay to play with your own boobs, even when you are breastfeeding. What are the other things you love that your partner can do for your body?

Madison: *Breastfeeding can sometimes also be accompanied by chapped nipples and soreness of breasts or nipples, which can make the idea of having one's breasts touched seem unappealing. Any tips on navigating around these issues?*

Moorea: *It is common for breastfeeding to hurt, but it really shouldn't. Cracked nipples or pain often suggest that there is a problem with the baby's latch that could be corrected. The breastfeeding parent should definitely attempt to get as much lactation help as possible from an IBCLC (International Board Certified Lactation Consultant)—she is the boob's best friend. In the meantime, lanolin can prevent cracking. Earth Mama Angel Baby Natural Nipple Butter (which is lanolin free) is fantastic (and makes a good lube too!). Does it feel good for your partner to stroke or cup your breasts but not touch the nipples? Can your partner gently massage nipple butter into your breasts and nipples? Or do you need to negotiate* staying away from the breasts altogether until your body is more adjusted to breastfeeding? Talk before you get into the heat of the moment.

Some women report that the general heaviness of the breasts when they first begin breastfeeding is a turn-on, and some report it being uncomfortable. We must communicate our feelings and requests to our partners. Hot and cold are both good remedies for uncomfortable breasts. If a woman has a clogged duct or mastitis, she most likely does not feel like any breast play at all. She should consult an MD, ND, or lactation consultant, and both partners should try to be patient with breast play and know that the problem will resolve quickly with treatment.

Madison: I think one of the biggest challenges I faced postpartum was psychological. I felt like my body wasn't my own. Both because my body was being occupied so constantly by another creature and because it wasn't the body that I recognized as mine. It was in no way my pre-mom body, even though I was no longer carrying a child. It was a strange period of feeling engulfed in a huge transition without knowing what I was transitioning into. I remember breasts that were leaking and would shoot out milk when I'd laugh, one breast being a full cup size bigger than the other one, and my body not feeling like my own. What is your advice for loving our awkward postpartum bodies as they are in the moment? Any self-care advice on going through the transition?

Moorea: Such an excellent point! How unnerving to feel like our body is not our own! If we are nursing a young baby, it feels like we exist solely for the consumption of this new being. It helps to do things with our bodies that are *not about the baby, and sex or masturbation can actually be one of these, but another excellent way to love your postpartum body is to exercise it. I would suggest getting a workout specifically around other mother-bodies of all stages! Belly dance or Zumba classes are places moms frequent, as well as gyms that are geared less toward hard bodies and more toward moms and older people. The point is not to change your body or lose weight with an exercise program; it is to get you out of the house and raise your endorphins, which will make you feel sexier and help your mood! Another great way to learn to love your postpartum body is to be around other bodies that are dripping milk everywhere! This could be a postnatal exercise class, a mom's group, or a breastfeeding group. Mama-baby yoga class saved me in so many ways.*

New moms are so busy with holding babies that we tend to shower less. Try to make sure you are able to shower off the spit-up daily and have a moment to be with your body and your mind. Do take advantage of help. If you don't have a partner who can help with alone time, ask that neighbor who said he wanted to hold the baby. Just as with sex, ask for what you need, and receive with pleasure that which is being given to you.

Madison: *How do you recommend women reclaim their breasts while still breastfeeding? And how do we find the time to reclaim our breasts while in the midst of new motherhood?*

Moorea: *I think reclaiming our breasts is more about relearning consent and less about finding time. Reclaiming isn't really possible with a newborn—they actually kind of own your boobs. Now, having an older baby or toddler needing our breasts can confuse us a little regarding what* *we have learned about sharing our bodies only when we feel like it. I write a lot about this topic and I mention it to all of my sleep clients, especially when they are thinking about gradually night weaning. Since nursing on demand is the best way to start our babies out, we often continue this way and then begin to feel resentful if our child wants to nurse when we don't feel like it. I suggest beginning to model consent for your children early so they know it is okay to tell others "yes" and "no" about their own bodies! As soon as your child can understand yes and no and can use a first few words or signs, get in touch with your body each time your baby grabs for it and respond honestly with whether or not you want to share your body in this moment. You can always say "No. I don't feel like nursing now. Ask me again later/after lunch." You can offer a bite of solid food, water, or a hug instead.*

Being free (free from tantrums!) to nurse when you want to and not nurse when you don't is one of the main keys to reclaiming your body. I nursed my daughter for three and a half years, but in those last years I only nursed her when it was mutually agreeable.

A SEXY MAMA'S POV
WITH ANYA DE MONTIGNY

My son is currently twelve years old and the joy of my life.

I had a natural childbirth at Sage Femme Midwifery in San Francisco, and my plan was to attachment parent and breastfeed until we naturally weaned together.

When my son was around two years old, I had been up with him for most of the night for his whole life, and I was a total basket case trying to work part-time and keep our little family together through some tough transitions. A client, noticing how tired and spaced out I was, suggested that I begin the weaning process, and I decided to take her advice. I was getting two to six hours of sleep a night, and the on-demand style of breastfeeding I was doing was no longer fitting my lifestyle, my sanity, or my need for autonomy at work. On-demand nursing was not all I had hoped it would be, and child-led weaning was going to need some help from mom. So, I pushed the night weaning process along even faster than planned, and my son began sleeping in the other room with his dad while I got some desperately needed sleep in my own bed, alone. It was hard—my son didn't want to do it. However, he did get to bond with papa over a month-long period, and ultimately I believe that this was the right thing for them and their relationship, which is beautiful and healthy to this day.

Even though my reasons for weaning came from a place of self-care and self-love, when I eventually did wean completely, I felt that maybe I had made a mistake. I longed for the connection that nursing brought to my son and me.

I often think that we do not talk about the intimacy we get from nursing because it's a huge taboo in our culture. Even though it's gaining more popularity to nurse in public, it is still "under wraps" and under blankets, something that a lot of women want to do privately because it's still not safe or socially acceptable to nurse in public. The hormones that are released when nursing are similar to what we experience during lovemaking, and they can feel amazing in ways that love, sex, and deep intimacy can feel. Talking about this in communities of women, I believe, can be transformative to the ways in which we view intimacy in our bodies and the ways in which we allow pleasure to exist within our expressions of being mothers.

Losing this connection with my son was akin to losing a deep connection to a lover on an emotional and very physical level. For years and years after he was done nursing, my son would reach out to hold my breast, and oftentimes he did this in public, pushing his hand underneath my shirt and holding on while I carried him. I had no shame in this. This was a connection that we had established right from the start, and it felt like the least we could do once we had ended that special bond of nursing.

I kept a diary of all of the ups and downs of my pregnancy and my "attachment parenting" style, and I wrote an entry right after I stopped nursing completely. It describes a very intense, emotional, and tumultuous state of mind that I believe speaks to the dropping off of hormones and the identity issues, frustration, and emotions that come from ending such an intimate experience with one's child. I was in a state of such confusion about myself and my identity as a mother. For so long I had been attached body to body with this being, and I was now, as I described it, "alone in my body." Between the hormone changes and the identity changes, I was really struggling.

1/22/05

I am starting a new journey. My mind is crazed these days! My hormones are just raging with coming off nursing. I have been driving my family and myself crazy as well.

I am feeling so much, too much. Sometimes I just want to cry and rage. I get so angry these days. I think that I miss nursing. It was soothing and calming. It was, until the end, a beautiful reprieve from the stresses of life and the responsibilities of being a parent. I miss the hormonal rush, the feelings of ease and contentment, the unfolding of peace within my mind and my belly.

Without it, I am a raging beast. A cyclone of fear and anger that lashes out and lashes in. It's like I can't stop my mind from crashing upon itself like a trainwreck. I spin and spin in circles without a grounding point, without that moment when my body stops, stops all mental activity to just be, to nourish, to make all better, all well in the world to a little baby. It's a very alone feeling, this being so alone now in my body. I want to pull someone aside, anyone, and tell/share/scream all of this at them, because I need to know that I am not crazy...

Some days I think that I need medication. But, in all truth, these feelings are life, they are living, they are the highs of sensitivity that I have been blessed with as a healer and an artist. I am a real person and I am going to feel. If there is a higher purpose for me on this planet, I am finding it piece by piece, and these days the pieces are coming together so fast that I cannot see a picture emerging. I do trust that there is one.

The last paragraph speaks to questioning my identity as a woman in the world: If I am no longer attached to a baby "body to body" in a literal sense, what is my purpose? Do I still have one? Am I still of use to anyone? These questions eventually became resolved, in part, when the hormones finished shifting around and I became more settled in my body.

I believe that attachment parenting, co-sleeping, and extended nursing were the most important decisions I made as a radical mama committed to the work of women's sexual empowerment. I believe that although it can be hard to choose this path, it's ultimately the deepest connection we can maintain to the cycles of life, sexuality, birth, and death that are available to us as beings who birth.

I have the most intimate, loving, and holistic connection with my son, and now, a good ten years later after I wrote that journal entry, I feel that I am living the deepest purpose of my life as a sex educator, partner, and mother. I am truly blessed to have had such a real, raw, and marvelous experience during it all, and I believe that part of the reason why I stand up for women's sexual empowerment is that I've personally gone through it all—and come out the other side!

4

Navigating Partnered Sex during Pregnancy

I ALWAYS KNEW THAT my sexuality and sexual desire were fluid, but pregnancy brought about a tsunami of changes that were radically erratic in nature and had me constantly pausing to check in with what my body was craving in that moment. The way I navigated these erratic changes was by moving a bit more slowly from one sexual act to another and taking more time to negotiate with sexual partners.

Pre-Intimacy Check-In

Are you about to engage in some form of intimate connection with your partner? Ask yourself these quick check-in questions in order to identify the type of intimate connection and sexual adventure that might best suit your and your partner's needs on any given day, during your pregnancy or after.

1. What is my current energy level?
2. Are there parts of my body that are craving a certain type of touch right now?
3. Are there parts of my body that feel agitated or sore or have an aversion to touch right now?
4. Are there particular positions that are more comfortable for me than others right now?

Asking for What You Want

One of the most common challenges I hear from women about their sex lives is a discomfort with asking for what they want. This is not limited to pregnancy or parenthood, but can be challenging for all individuals. It can come up during pregnancy in particular, though, because your partner may think he or she knows what you like, having been with you for some time. But even as the person experiencing touch, you might not know what you like until you're in the thick of it because your body is changing so rapidly during pregnancy. So pregnant women need to be even more assertive in asking for what they want and giving honest feedback during sex.

Giving Feedback during Sex

- Try to give information with a passion for the positive rather than a focus on the negative. Example: "It feels so good when you slather my pussy with lots of lube. Mmm—more lube, please."
- Give adjustments with praise. Example: "Your lips feel so good on my nipples. You're getting me so wet. I want to feel your hands on my cunt. Yes. More fingers. Harder, please."
- Try begging. Example: "Oh, please fill me up with your cock. Now slow, please! Yes, my love. Oh God, I want you to pump in and out of me nice and slow while you're spanking my ass. Oh yes. Oh please. I want it so bad. I want to come for you so bad."

Exercise: Energy Boost

It's not unusual to feel a dip in energy during pregnancy—especially in the first trimester. Give yourself an energy boost by moving your body. Stand up with your feet a little more than hip-width apart. Now, start to sway from side to side. It's great if you can do this exercise in your bare feet and really connect your body to the earth. Allow all the orgasmic, pulsing pleasure from each individual that is breathing in the room, in the house, in the neighborhood, in your city, in your state, your country— from every individual that is experiencing pleasure and ecstasy around the globe—to infuse your vessel with its radiant ecstatic energy.

Start to undulate your hips in circles, taking that pleasure, that energy, that ecstasy and swirling it around your pelvic region in small and large circles, experimenting with size, stirring the energy around. Imagine this thick and juicy, red-hot and orange sticky molten flowing energy that stretches and spins its way around your core, your heart, your throat, spouting out the top of your head. Using your deep inhales and exhales, moan and release this energy while simultaneously calling out into the world for a never-ending flow and cycle of more energy to run through your body. Energy and ecstasy from the world around you, spouting upward like a geyser from the earth, up your feet and legs, finding the immense power between your legs. You can growl and howl and moan and release deep-bellied breaths as the rainbow of colors and pleasure reaches from the crown of your head out past the roof, out into the night, out to the stars and the moon, embracing and stimulating the stars and planets in the deep beyond, embracing the universe in the strength of your powerful pleasure and energy. Let out an animalistic deep-body howl, purr, or meow.

Slowly start to slow your breath and return to a slow swaying of your body, back and forth. Shake your body. Bring your hands to your heart and feel how open it is, allowing loving energy to gently pulse and massage your insides. If your eyes are closed, now is a great time to open them and slowly, in your own time, find your way back to your grounding. Back to here and now. Full of love and energy.

Intimacy Exercise: Connected by Touch, Connected by Words

Sit across from your partner. Have ready a small object such as a ball, a rock, a crystal, a stick—any object that you can pass back and forth easily. I feel that more natural, less synthetic objects carry the energy back and forth with greater ease, but you can experiment and see what works best for you.

Both you and your partner should be sitting cross-legged and facing one another. Your bodies can be very close, so that your legs are actually touching one another. Start by holding the passing object to your heart and breathing with it several times—deep inhales and exhales. Upon exhale, when you are ready, place the object into your partner's hands, allowing your hands to touch. Both your hands and your partner's are touching each other and the object. Stay here for an inhale and exhale or two, keeping eye contact and exhaling love. When your partner receives the object, he or she should bring it to his or her heart and inhale the love and energy and connection that you have passed on, feeling that energy in his or her body.

Go slow with this. Go slow with your breath. Breathe deeply. Really feel the energy between you and your partner. Really infuse your object with energy. Cultivate that intimate energy inside yourself. Feel your whole body inhaling and exhaling, contracting and expanding, actively receiving breath and energy and connection and giving it outwardly to your partner. As you receive this energy, know that you deserve love. Accept this energy and connection as a gift that you are worthy of and that you can transform into more love and compassion that swells inside of you and that you will send outward to the world and your partner.

Once you start to really feel the richness and connection of this exercise, you can add another layer. This time, when you exhale and hand off the object, say a loving affirmation to your partner, such as "You have beautiful eyes." Or "The curve of your ass is so sexy." Or "Your capacity to love others is inspiring." When your partner accepts and takes in this exhale, this affirmation, this object close to his or her heart, he or she will breathe with it, accept this affirmation, and state the affirmation back. "My eyes are beautiful." "The curve of my ass is sexy." "My capacity to love others is inspiring." After this reflection, your partner will pass the object back to you, with more love, affection, and energy. Your partner will exhale an affirmation to you while passing the object into your hands. You will want to do this several times back and forth.

Sexual Practices by Trimester

First trimester—This trimester is possibly the most difficult for many people. It often includes symptoms such as nausea and vomiting, heartburn, and total exhaustion, as well as breast and nipple soreness. Listen to your body and try not to push past what your body is telling you it needs. When my body was tired, I learned to take a nap. If I felt discomfort in my uterus when I leaned over someone's knee for a spanking, I just adjusted myself to another position. For the most part, I avoided impact around my abdomen. I engaged in safer-sex practices and didn't take any impact around my abdomen and uterus.

I was very lucky, as I didn't experience very much nausea during pregnancy, only heartburn. My libido was full force in my first trimester, and I really enjoyed sex during this time in my pregnancy. My breasts were really sore and so were my nipples, so that was something I had to consistently communicate to my partners. It also put nipple clamps, which I generally loved, onto my NO list for the first trimester.

Both for performance and in my personal sex life, rope suspension and rope bondage were something I greatly enjoyed. I had a wonderful sex-positive OB-GYN, and I was able to communicate openly with her about my work and my personal sex preferences in order to get honest, open, non-judgmental medical advice. I had asked my OB-GYN if rope bondage and rope suspension would be safe during the pregnancy, and she said absolutely. She said I wasn't a high-risk pregnancy, and that baby and I would be fine engaging in suspension through at least the first trimester and modified rope bondage throughout the pregnancy. This was my personal experience as someone who was well practiced at rope suspension for over ten years. I wouldn't advise someone who has never tried rope suspension to begin this practice during pregnancy. In Chapter 21 we talk about this topic with much more depth.

Second trimester—My breasts now felt wonderful and had blossomed into these erogenous curves that I'd never experienced before. I just wanted to keep playing with them. I loved breasts, and I now had them. I had never envisioned that this would happen. I kid you not, my cunt took on the sweet smell of cookies. In the second trimester, I was a nymphomaniac! I loved sex and felt like the ultimate powerful, pregnant sexual goddess. I wanted to be worshipped. My hair was lush and full and beautiful. My breasts were plump and round and begging for touch. All of my body parts that were swelling felt engorged and aroused and needing to be touched, kissed, and caressed. I couldn't masturbate or fuck enough. I just couldn't. I was insatiable.

Experts advise that you not lie on your back during the second and third trimesters. Lying on your back at this time can put additional pressure on the inferior vena cava, which can reduce blood flow to the placenta— so missionary position is out of the picture. However, you can use lots of pillows and prop yourself upright. There are also "sex wedges," which can be very helpful during pregnancy in finding a position that is comfortable for you. Some of the most popular ones are made by Liberator.

Above all, you want to be checking in with your body. How do you feel? When I started feeling a pressure and heaviness in my uterus in my second trimester, my mama instinct really shifted into full gear. I didn't want to be placed in a suspension in which rope would be pressing tightly against my uterus. My body was changing and I was no longer an athlete pushing my own body to its limits and extremes, but a guide, vessel, and protector for a new little person. I was still able to engage in many of the dominant and submissive kinks that I enjoyed, but I modified them to fit my changing body.

In the second trimester your circulation really changes. Moving from lying down to a standing position quickly, as might happen in some sexual situations, can make you dizzy. Also, constriction of the limbs can limit blood flow to the fetus, so you want to avoid tight bondage. I still enjoyed face slapping and hair pulling (both giving and receiving), service, role play, even nipple play in the second trimester. My nipples were back in action after being wildly sensitive during the first trimester. As a submissive (or even just when I'm giving oral sex), I enjoy being on my knees. This actually became a little problematic during the second trimester. I would lose circulation very easily from being in the same position for a while and would need to move to a more comfortable position. Adding pillows or blankets under my knees was helpful, as was sitting with my legs to the side of my body. Another thing to try might be a seated position with legs in front. Experiment with your body and find what works for you.

Spooning, cowgirl, and reverse cowgirl were also excellent positions during this time. For me, massage and sensual experiences or experiences that allowed me to exude more of my dominant side from being on top were the most satisfying at this point in my pregnancy. I would experience some discomfort occasionally and would need to move to accommodate my growing pregnant body. Another thing I hadn't really expected was that my round belly became an extension of my vulva, a round, swollen, sensitive erogenous zone that loved to be massaged, lubricated, and touched. What new erogenous zones will you discover? Where does it feel good to be touched?

Third trimester—By my third trimester I was big! Big and beautiful. My joints and ligaments had really started to loosen with the release of a hormone known as relaxin. Our bodies start to do this in order to get our hips nice and loose and flexible and wide so our wee one can pass through the vaginal canal. As someone who was already quite flexible and who liked to do things like contortion, bondage, aerial performance, and yoga, I found that when I got to this point in the pregnancy—especially the last month—that I had to bring a great deal of consciousness to my body.

Even walking in heels or up hills became really problematic. I can't say that at thirty-six weeks I felt very sexy. My skin felt tight, like my body was going to rip in two, and I constantly felt like I was going to topple over. I didn't like feeling weaker than I had been in the second trimester. But I continued to enjoy masturbation. At this point, doggie-style, standing doggie-style, and spooning were the most comfortable. I also really enjoyed masturbating with a "vibe sandwich"—my body and vulva on one side, the bed or wedge on the other side, and a vibrator in the middle. This is also when a lot of stretch marks like to appear due to so much stretching of the skin, and it felt incredibly erotic to rub vitamin E oil blends on my belly and breasts.

Finding clothes that make you feel sexy can do wonders for your sexual confidence! You don't have to spend a lot. Look for clothes that are stretchy or flowing. Try going to secondhand shops and shopping outside of the maternity section for flowing and stretchy dresses or oversized blouses that are silky or feel really good next to your skin. What fabrics feel sexy and sensual to you? For me, thrift-store silky slips and stretchy evening gowns were pretty much all I was wearing toward the end of my pregnancy. I had one pair of pregnancy heels, which I got as I was entering the third trimester and started to experience some back pain. My pregnancy heels had a wider heel and greater arch support.

These days are to be treasured. This is a wonderful time to really savor silence, time by yourself, and intimacy with your partner. It's not like you'll never have time alone with your partner again, but negotiating that time alone becomes a lot more complicated after baby arrives.

As your pregnancy is nearing its end, think of this as a beautiful opportunity to build a whole new level of romance and intimacy with your partner. You're not the only one going through a transition. Your partner is going through a transition too, and the two of you are going through a transition together. Take time to gaze at the stars with your partner. Go on picnics. Lie in bed together naked making out and talking about your dreams, your future, and what you love about one another. Try cooking classes together, go to the museum, walk on the beach— don't forget to date and woo one another. May the love letters never stop. May the flowers be ever flowing. May your heart always race when your eyes meet from across a room.

A SEXY MAMA'S POV
WITH CAROLINE RHAME

The act of growing a human inside my body and getting it out was a massive experience for me. My first pregnancy was filled with fear over the impending birth and rage at my husband for not embracing my pregnant form the way I had expected. The idea of bringing a new life into the world was an anxiety-provoking concept for him. Anxiety plus my fast-changing body equaled zero sexual energy coming from my partner, from whom I'd been acclimated to receiving a healthy income of attraction. Rage, incidentally, also turned out to put a damper on our usual sexual heat.

At the end of my second trimester, I had bloody discharge from my left nipple. A bit alarmed, I proceeded through a stream of doctors and screenings and allowed myself to be pressured into an unnecessary breast surgery that removed a golf ball–sized amount of healthy breast tissue from behind my nipple. The healing process in my third trimester was slow and brutal, and the nipple was much changed from its previous state. My primary concerns centered on whether I'd be able to breastfeed from it, as well as straight-up vanity.

The outcome was that I wasn't be able to breastfeed from that side, I had a newly altered breast that I would need to accept and fall in love with, and I had a fresh supply of white-hot napalm anger with which I was ready to decimate. My husband was a daisy in my crosshairs, and I railed at him.

Thirty-eight hours into labor, I lay bedraggled in a hospital bed. After the medical violation of my breast, I snarled at every physician, resident, or nurse who broached the topic of a C-section with me. I cleared the room and for the first time allowed myself to be alone with my baby. I saw her wanting to come out, and I saw her moving down with each contraction.

Less than an hour later, I miraculously had a perfect child in my arms. I was shocked by her sheer individuality. She was a complete stranger who I would have taken a bullet for within five minutes of knowing her. I forgave my husband, and I forgave myself. I grabbed my breasts every morning and told them that I loved them.

For the second preggo go-round, I was braced for the withdrawal of sexual heat that had returned with a vengeance after the first birth. I knew it would come back, and I fully indulged in self-pleasuring. The increased blood volume and the rise in hormones made me a little red-hot engine of horniness both times. I captured my energy the second time and rode it every day.

I looked forward to a more relaxed experience at a birthing center. I knew that I was tipping into labor on that January morning. I kept it to myself in the way that is sometimes required to maintain magic. I shut my bedroom door and self-pleasured. Once again I sought to be alone with my baby. I took my time. I didn't expedite my orgasm with a vibrator, but instead used my slow hand to seduce my body and my labor.

That morning I used my mind's eye to see my second daughter move through me with perfect alignment. I sent an invitation to my body to surrender. She was born seven hours later without a fight.

We've all heard that the mind's ability to visualize is everything when it comes to birth. I agree wholeheartedly. I would also extrapolate that concept and give it a turbo-charge from the act of self-pleasuring. It works. Visualization combined with pleasure pulls everything you want into sharp relief. It lines up the world to serve you. Whether it's your dream house you're bidding on, a job you're interviewing for, or bringing a life into this world, anger and fear are hitched—and pleasure and the courting of what you want are inextricably linked.

5

Sleep

SLEEP. OH, DEAR SLEEP. Where have you gone? Sometimes the idea of sleep sounds so much sweeter than the idea of sex! The intimacy of sleeping alone with your partner in bed, in a house or a hotel by yourselves, can sound so much more connected and precious and intimate than an orgasm. When enduring the challenges of sleep deprivation, an uninterrupted night of sleep can seem orgasmic. Our bodies need sleep. We need it. It's essential for our survival, and yet as new parents, we walk into a zombie minefield of sleeplessness.

Sometimes it's more challenging for certain babies and parents to find sleep than for others. My little one had colic and had a very challenging time sleeping anywhere but my chest—which meant I didn't sleep for about a year. I'm sure that my first wrinkles were a result of that year of sleeplessness. Sleep is a huge factor in our well-being, our partner's well-being, and our child's well-being. It also greatly factors into our emotional state of being, our relationships, our communication, and the intimacy and connection that we feel with our partner and child.

INTERVIEW WITH MOOREA MALATT
PARENTING COACH AND
SLEEP SAVVY EXPERT

Madison: *When people aren't sleeping, they aren't generally feeling very sexy. Perhaps one of the greatest immediate changes in my life going into motherhood was a dramatic reduction in the amount of sleep that was happening in the house. What have you discovered about the way that lack of sleep affects libido and sexual intimacy between partners?*

Moorea: *Sleep deprivation can kill your sex life for a while, and rats that get as small an amount of sleep as new human mothers do actually die of sleep deprivation. Human lactation hormones, though, are somehow protective of our mama brains! Many moms who love breastfeeding still think breastfeeding through the night sucks. Breastfed babies do wake more frequently because they drink less at one feed, because breast milk is easier and faster to digest than formula, and because we were set up biologically to wake to keep our mothers out of a deep sleep so that they can hear other animals coming and protect us. Though we still wake more frequently, breastfeeding moms report being more rested than formula-feeding moms of new babies—possibly because they may be co-sleeping, nursing in bed, and not getting out of bed at all at night.*

Sleep deprivation causing mom to be too tired for sex may have evolved for child spacing the way breastfeeding's delaying of menstruation has. Knowing a possible reason we have to wake so many times at night doesn't really help our sex life, though! Mom's partner is often also very sleep deprived, and there is very little time left for connecting because tired moms go to bed much earlier, get up much earlier, and hopefully are napping when the baby naps. It is can be virtually impossible for a man to get it up when he is very sleep deprived. Napping during the day when the baby sleeps so that you have a little reserve for your partner at night is a great idea, even if you can only afford to do this once on the weekend.

Madison: How does lack of sleep affect communication among partners? What tools do you recommend to strengthen communication between partners during this lack of sleep that new parents experience?

Moorea: This is the best question. If you have never even fought before, this will likely be the time. Lack of sleep in parenting can either make parents edgy and blaming, or bring them together because they are experiencing the same little hell. When things get tense, I recommend saying "This new job is so hard for me. Share with me the ways it is hard for you." Sometimes the sleep deprivation can make us actually feel crazy, and we say mean things. If things feel really bad, ask your partner, "Are we partners in parenting or enemies?" It's a drastic question that can shift perspective on the little things. You can bring a baby to couples therapy or solo therapy with some specialists who who specialize in life cycle adjustments. I did it.

With regard to sex and communication, I think the breastfeeding mama should communicate with herself first—really make a point of getting to know her new body, appreciating it, and using it in non-baby ways, and also talking to her partner about this new breastfeeding body. It is just like when I teach gentle discipline and kids are stealing toys. Developmentally, we have to know what it is to own something before we can learn how to share it. It is hard to want to have sex when we are worried about what will happen during the act, how things currently feel to our body, or what our partner thinks about our body. Own it, know it, then talk about it and share your insecurities.

Madison: *Many parents I know end up sleeping in separate beds due to mother/child co-sleeping, night nursing, etc., especially if one is in need of sleep to function for work the next day. I know this can create feelings of being replaced, or a fracture in the connection and intimacy between partners. Any suggestions on how to keep the mother/child bond and intimacy but also make room for partner bonding and intimacy? How do you suggest that parents make room and space for intimate and sexual time together while co-sleeping?*

Moorea: *So many families sleep in separate beds so that one partner can get more sleep and baby can still co-sleep and nurse. I did it this way myself with a double bed in the baby's room instead of a crib. It is a practical way of life (mirrored by some indigenous cultures where the men sleep separately from the women), but it doesn't mean sex goes out the window. You just have to stop thinking about sex as a bed activity. Intimate time can be caught in the shower, in the middle of the day on a weekend during the baby's nap, in the kitchen. Let your two hours of date night be tacos and car sex instead of a restaurant.*

Partners often just miss having that before-bed couple time, even if it isn't about sex. It really helps co-sleeping families if mom can put baby to bed in the co-sleeping room and sneak out for an hour to snuggle with her sweetie. The non-nursing parent can also lie in the co-sleeping bed for family togetherness just during the time that the baby is nursing to sleep, and then both parents can sneak out for adult time.

Madison: What tips do you suggest for parents in terms of obtaining the sleep and self-care they need to nourish their relationship with each other and have the energy they need for intimate connection and sexual pleasure?

Moorea: I wish we could all do parenting as a village, instead of taking on every task and pressure between one or two parents. Stress is not conducive to feeling sexy. Ask for help and then ask for more help. Ask grandparents, friends, neighbors to help with household chores or with the baby—don't just wait for them to offer. Find a way to get a date night and use it for intimacy. Can you afford a house cleaner? It's easier to feel sexy when housework isn't staring at you. If your sleep situation is really bad, you may want to hire a postpartum doula or a sleep coach (I say find a gentle attachment and breast-feeding–based one, but then, I'm biased!) so that one day you may just be rested enough to get it on.

The most important tip is to be gentle and understanding and respectful to one another as new parents, in the same way you are gentle to your baby. Pressure to have sex, being grabbed at, being constantly asked if you are ready, and being guilt-tripped about not having the energy are all turn-offs.

A SEXY MAMA'S POV
WITH ASHLEY PIA

Becoming pregnant is the most amazing transition, physically, mentally, but in my case especially sexually. I've been with my partner now for ten years, but it was only when I became pregnant that things changed, and it was a learning experience. My sexuality has always been a driving force in who I am. I'm a romantic, a lover, and a giver in every sense of the word. I've always had a healthy sex life, but everything changed for me twelve weeks into my pregnancy.

It was time to find out the sex of the baby, and I couldn't have been more excited. Shortly after the doctor had announced it was indeed a girl (as I had known from the beginning) and I had left the doctor's office, my phone rang. "Mrs. Pia, I have some news, and it's serious," the doctor said. I had a condition, and I couldn't have intercourse or do anything strenuous for the rest of my pregnancy. I felt as though I had hit a brick wall and my breath had been knocked out of me. My concern was for my daughter, of course, but I also felt a sense of loss. I felt full and voluptuous and radiant and powerful, and I couldn't have sex...hmmmmm.

My first call was to my partner, who was only concerned about me and told me it wasn't a big deal as long as I was safe and healthy. My mother chimed in and said, "There's always BJs and other stuff you can do!" with her supportive mom smile.

I lay down a few nights later and started to kiss my partner. I hadn't felt so aroused by kissing in a long time. It was soft and slow, and because, in the back of my mind,

I knew we couldn't have sex, I savored it. We made out for what seemed like hours, and I almost climaxed just from kissing. This was new and very surprising. We started exploring each other's bodies, spending hours massaging, caressing, sucking, and kissing each other's necks, mouths, backs, legs, and shoulders. It was a celebration of our bodies in a new way, and it was more intimate then we had ever been. It was these sweet, slow kisses all over my body that really connected me to my partner and gave me a sense of pleasing him because he enjoyed it so much. We explored areas in more detail, and it breathed a whole new essence into our love life.

I had never physically been so large, but I had also never felt so beautiful. We continued the other usual activities. But for me, the true intimacy was this buried hidden treasure that we found together. In a time of taking something away, we gained so much more.

After my amazing daughter was born, I entered a state of bliss, because I had this tiny human who I loved more than anything. On the other hand, I was left with a body that I didn't recognize and that wasn't cooperating with me. I had stretch marks and extra skin, and I was tired and worn out because sleep was a luxury I no longer got to enjoy when I wanted. I was pushing myself to lose weight but wasn't seeing results, and I was being very hard on myself.

My family told me that it took time and that my body would never be just like before baby, but it was hard to hear. I was beyond happy with my daughter, but depressed about my body. I was crying every day and everything made me emotional. It was crazy to feel like I had no control over my emotions, but here's a little fact I found out: It can take a year or more for your hormones to balance out after baby.

I started to slowly lose some extra weight and embrace and love my new body. It was a yearlong process of making smarter eating choices and walking and taking the stairs instead of the elevator. My body is not what it was before, and I'm okay with that.

My partner and I have a bond now that we never had before. Maybe because we worshipped each other in our rawness during my pregnancy, or because we are raising a child we made, or the years we've spent with each other, or all of it.

The truth is, pregnancy changed me for the better. It was a growing experience and remains that way.

Creating a Sexual Empowerment
Manifesto, Finding Time for Sex

A MANIFESTO IS AN open and powerful declaration of who you are. It is unapologetic. It is celebratory and empowering. A manifesto embodies all the best parts of who you are and who you will be. It can have a specific focus and embody one particular aspect of your life, such as a feminist manifesto, a mothering manifesto, an earth as lover manifesto, or a submissive's manifesto. It is a promise to yourself. Not expectations, but a pillar of strength that will fill your vessel with the energy and encouragement that you need to persevere when you feel weak and to embrace the life you want to live. A manifesto provides the inspiration you need to manifest the life you truly desire.

I've included my own sexual empowerment manifesto here to get your sexy mama creative juices flowing.

Madison Young's Sexual Empowerment Manifesto

I am fierce and powerful. I embody sexual power from my toes to the crown of my head and everywhere in between. My sexual desire and expression is not dependent on my partner; my desire is mine and mine alone. I will fuck my desire. I will fuck with my desire. I will shapeshift into multiple forms and different bodies like a mystical creature. My cunt is hungry and powerful; it devours everything it touches—cocks, hands, fists, dildos. It is ravenous. My anus is starving and all-

consuming, ecstatic to the touch—epicenter of my erotic power, my root chakra, pulsing, aching, radiating with a powerful desire for touch, for sensation, for love, for compassion. I will be your nourishment and you will be mine; devour me whole and I will eat you from the inside, heart first, and then birth you, my dear, my love, all over again. We will engulf one another, overcome with pleasure like the epic waves of the Pacific Ocean that I love to dance in and run through like a child. I will be your little girl and your slut. I will be my own hero. I will celebrate my sexual radiance with every moon, with every drop of rain that falls upon my skin, with every brilliant ray of light that streams from the morning sky.

In order to manifest the life you desire to live—and the sex life you desire—you must first visualize what that might look like.

Before we sketch out our manifestos, let's solidify the vision of our sex lives that we want to manifest. Grab a bunch of magazines and tear out words and images that embody your vision of your sexy mama sex life. Don't feel limited to traditionally "sexy" images. It doesn't have to be a bunch of images of Victoria's Secret models in lingerie. What images and words appeal to your sensual being? What images warm your heart and make you feel giddy with excitement? Pictures of cupcakes? Waves crashing on the shore? Towering redwood trees? A pair of leather boots? A photo of a woman reading a book? Try not to judge or censor yourself. All of these subjects can inform your sex life, sexual adventures, or fantasies that you may wish to explore. Did you tear out pictures of a serene beach or pool setting? Sex on the beach or underwater blow jobs in a swimming pool can be a blast! Did you tear out images of a bookshelf full of books? Are you a bibliophile? Do books turn you on? Try reading erotica to your partner at night, or reading your partner's favorite book while you receive a spanking! Turned on by cupcakes? Become a delicious sweet delight for your partner and try having him or her eat a cupcake from between your breasts. Yum! Maybe you plucked out a photo from National Geographic of a howling wolf or a prowling tiger? Follow your animal instinct. These spirit animals can inspire and inform your sexual identity in a primal way.

Choose images that appeal to you and then examine what it is about them that you love, or what appeals to you emotionally and sexually.

Assemble them on a vision board or inspiration board (let's call it your sexy mama vision board). Keep this above your desk, in your bedroom, or somewhere you will see it each day. Within these images, you will find clues to the manifesto you desire. Based on your vision board, what do you envision when you think of your sexy mama sex life?

Take a moment to consider the images that you picked out, their significance, and the erotic path they might suggest for you in your sexy mama sex life. In what way do these images appeal to your sensual and sexual nature? How do the images affect you emotionally and energetically? Do you feel inspired? At peace? Tranquil? Ravenous? Ferocious? Fierce? Carnal and animalistic? Playful? Where in your body do you feel these emotions and energies stirring? Linger with those feelings for a while. Lie back, close your eyes, and allow yourself to step into these images, these worlds. What fantasies unfold for you? Remember, there is no judgment. Try to explore the environment in your fantasy with all of your senses. What do you feel against your skin? What parts of your body are you exploring the fantasy world with? Your mouth? Your eyes? Your feet? What do you smell? What sounds do you hear?

This type of guided visualization exercise allows you to flex your imagination and spark desire. It gives you permission to explore the real world with your whole body, with all of your senses. When we start to truly explore the world energetically and sexually—not just with our genitals, but allowing ourselves to lean deeply into the pleasure of small moments of connection, touch, and sensation—our erotic selves become supercharged and awakened, even when we might be totally exhausted from late nights with a colicky infant.

In the Chaos of Motherhood, How Do I Find My Sexual Empowerment?

You might be thinking, "Yeah, thanks, Madison. When exactly am I going to find all this time to create a vision board, or have two seconds to think about my sex life? I haven't showered in two days, and my dishes are piled up in the sink!"

I hear you. When I first entered into motherhood, I asked one of my friends, who gave birth to her second child on the same day that I gave birth to my first child, "How do you do it? You seem so calm! I feel like a frazzled mess. How do you juggle all these balls and not let anything drop?"

What she said totally changed my perspective and truly was one of the simplest and greatest early parenting gems of wisdom that I received. She said "Oh, the balls drop. They drop all the time. But I know they are going to drop and I choose which is going to drop and I'm okay with it. I drop different balls on different days and I just let it go and move on." Said with the true confidence of a second-time mother!

This helped me to realize that I needed to choose and cycle through what I was prioritizing on different days. If I struggled to excel at everything every day, I only felt like a failure. Certain things needed my undivided attention and would suffer if I tried to multitask. Sometimes what I needed was to make a vision board and meditate—and sometimes I needed this more than I needed a shower! Sometimes having sex in the kitchen while our child was napping was more important than tending to the dirty dishes. But sometimes doing the dishes while your partner sexually stimulates you can be a fun way to get chores done. In fact, it's probably my favorite way to do dishes.

Another mom told me that the greatest thing she did to take care of herself postpartum was to have a teenage neighbor come over for an hour every night and take the baby for a stroll around the block while she and her husband had dinner (and sometimes sex!) alone in the apartment. It was only an hour, so it didn't cost much, but it was a way that she and her husband were able to connect intimately every night. It's crucial for us to fill our vessels. To care for ourselves. We might not be able to do everything we used to in the same way that we used to, but getting creative is the name of the game when it comes to parenting and intimacy.

Sometimes what we need sexually is alone time. In fact, often a major contributing factor to a decreased libido is that new moms are needed twenty-four seven and are being touched and fed on by another person all day long. Your privacy essentially goes out the window. Being around another individual constantly—especially when they need you and depend on you for everything—can leave little to no space for your own emotions, your own needs, your own body.

A couple at one of my workshops, who had a child under a year old, asked me a question after class. The husband worked all day, and the mom had decided to stay home and take care of their child for the first couple of years. The husband said to me, "In your class you talk about a flow of energy and intimacy back and forth from one body to another, from one vessel to another, but I feel like I have all this sexual energy that I'm putting out, and I'm not getting anything back from my wife." When I heard this, I smiled and exhaled, knowing that the husband loved his wife and desperately wanted the same intimacy and connection that they had experienced prior to the birth of their child. I explained to him, "If your wife's vessel is empty—void of energy—because she has been tending to someone else's needs all day, she will likely experience difficulty in reciprocating or even really receiving the sexual energy that you are putting forth. Her vessel is empty. She needs self-care, space, and time to get to a nourished, healthy space before she can truly start to cultivate desire within herself to share with her husband."

Sometimes one of the greatest things a partner can do for you is to let you sleep, or feed the baby a bottle in the middle of the night so you don't have to get up, or take the baby for a stroll to give you time to take a yoga class on your own or a relaxing bath. Even an hour of recharging time can be so nourishing, and the more often you can build in regular time for nourishment, the healthier and more energetic you are likely to feel.

Exercise: Clear the Guilt

You deserve to be nourished and loved! Get out a pen and paper, and for five minutes, just purge all of those voices, excuses, expectations, and judgments that might be blocking you from engaging in the nourishment and self-care that you deserve. This doesn't have to be complete sentences, or even make sense to anyone but you. This is for you. Write it all down, and then look it over, tear it up, and burn it. Release all that negative energy and judgment. Let it all go. Clear the way for the love you deserve to enter your life. It's time to let your vessel fill and overflow.

Now, identify a few nourishing actions that you can incorporate into your daily life to nourish your vessel. Here are mine:

- Putting on red lipstick. My red lipstick is a power item for me. Even if I have no time to shower or wash my hair, I can always muster ten seconds to put on my red lipstick, and it makes me feel better the whole day through.
- Wearing perfume. A warm, comforting vanilla scent, or amber, or one of my other favorite perfumes or essential oils, lifts me up through the day and keeps my senses awake.
- Putting on my ruby slippers. I always have a pair. The bright pop of color turns me on and feels empowering.
- Touching flowers. I love to stop and feel the flowers, rub the bark on a tree, walk barefoot through the grass. Pick flowers, grow flowers, buy yourself flowers.
- Looking outside and saying goodnight to the moon.
- Playing my favorite songs that I can belt out and dance around the house to. Music is wildly stimulating and inspiring, and can really get your body moving.

Next, identify the time or times of the day when you most need that nourishment. For me I find this is first thing in the morning, then around three o'clock or so, and also late at night before bed when I'm decompressing from the day. These are times when I am often either hungry or tired. Just as our children can be prickly and need a little extra love and nourishment when they are hungry or tired, so can we. Keeping snacks with me and having music handy to lift me up when I need a pick-me-up—and coffee or tea—is all part of my self-care and nourishment routine. When do you need a little extra help? What times of the day? What are ways that you can address those feelings and make life a little simpler during those times so you can fuel your vessel? I'm a huge fan of working out a trade with other parents. Do you need a night alone with your husband? Trade sleepovers. Your kid sleeps over at a friend's house one weekend, and the next weekend you take their kids. Need time to jog, do yoga, or work on your latest art project? Trade time with a friend—you take the kids for three hours in the morning and have your friend take them for three hours in the afternoon.

Okay, now that you know what you need and when you need it, put it on the calendar. Do you need a long luxurious bubble bath once a week? Or a soak in a hot tub? Or a massage? Or yoga? Whatever it is, put it on the calendar and figure out the logistics of childcare. Now you're committed. Just like you put dentist's and doctor's appointments on the calendar, you're going to put your weekly mani/pedi on there, too, and develop a routine that incorporates self-care. Caring for yourself is also caring for your sexual self and for your intimate relationship with your partner. Remember, if your vessel isn't full, there won't be anything to give to your partner, friends, or child. Taking care of yourself is taking care of your family.

Make a list of all the things that occupy your life right now and the percentage of your time that they take up, and take a look at the list. Are sex, pleasure, and self-care on the list? If not, add them and give them a percentage. Does the list reflect the amount of your time that you want to be giving to those parts of your life? Here's an example:

Mothering/household: 77.5 percent
Work: 15 percent
Time with partner: 3 percent
Self-care: 2 percent
Community events and time with friends: 1 percent
Sex and kink: 1 percent
Financial management: 0.5 percent

Now, create another list. Your dream list. What things do you want to have occupying your life, and what percentage of your time would you like to spend on each of those areas of your life?

Mothering/household: 55 percent
Work: 15 percent
Creative pursuits: 10 percent
Self-care: 5 percent
Sex and kink: 5 percent
Time with partner: 5 percent

Community events and time with friends: 4 percent

Financial management: 1 percent

How do you feel, looking at that dream list of how you want to spend your time? Where do you need to make shifts in your schedule? What do you need to do to manifest those changes? What support might you need? Trading childcare with a friend so you can have date nights? Bringing in a sitter so you can spend more time writing or making art or going to yoga? Fitting in a manicure once a month, as opposed to the once a week that you were able to fit in pre-motherhood?

Repeat after me:

> *I deserve to live my dream. I am capable of manifesting the life I desire. I am capable of change. I am evolving and I am perfect as I am in this moment. I deserve love. I deserve pleasure. I deserve connection. I deserve to fill my vessel with love and adoration. I am releasing any pain and shame surrounding the idea of caring for myself. In caring for myself, I am caring for my children and the people in my life that I love.*

TIPS ON CULTIVATING SELF-LOVE AND COMPASSION
WITH NATASHIA FUKSMAN, MA

Take time for self-care on a daily or weekly basis. It doesn't have to be something out of your price range. It can be your walk each week, your hot bath at night, your cup of tea before everybody else wakes up. Develop some kind of rhythm of self-care time, taking some of that time to find grounding within yourself, and some of that time to find grounding with others—not just one person. Find a community that includes other members, like a partner, of course, but also other women who are in or around the same stage of motherhood.

Find regular self-care time—both individual and with the greater community—that is focused on some sort of internal grounding process. Some people will have women's groups or a spiritual community; some people will take time every day to look at their body; some people will masturbate every day, or every week. Find something that will give back to your own soul.

A SEXY MAMA'S POV
WITH CARLIN ROSS

When you're forty-one and pregnant, you don't know how your body is going to rebound after giving birth. I left most of my spring and summer dresses in storage because I didn't know how long it would take to lose the weight. I listened to the admonitions of my mother and my friends, who warned that it took six to twelve months to get your body back. Somehow I thought I'd still be in maternity wear for several months and then sweats for the rest of the year.

I simply didn't have an image of my post-pregnancy body. And I assumed the worst because of my age. Yes, I only gained fourteen pounds, but what about skin elasticity and muscle loss and a stretched-out uterus? They say it's harder to get back in shape when you're older. I'd waited to start a family until my career was established and I'd had my fun—now I was going to pay.

These were my pre-labor thoughts. Post-labor was a different story. The one positive of my C-section was that the pain kept me focused on the present. I didn't give a rat's ass what I looked like. Everything was a challenge. The gym seemed a million miles away. This Friday will be my six-week checkup, and I'm finally able to move around pain-free. I finally feel like me again.

My first two weeks home from the hospital were a breastfeeding blur. My son is a cluster feeder, so he just keeps nursing. And we're sleep sharing because I couldn't get in and out of bed post-surgery. (Grayson sleeps across my chest. I have a pillow under one arm with his head nestled on me.) When you sleep share, you double the amount of daily feedings because your baby nurses all night.

Reading about babies nursing every three hours breaks me up—I nurse for three hours with an hour-long break in between. Let's just say that by his two-week well visit, Grayson gained back all the weight he lost coming home from the hospital, plus another two pounds.

What no one told me is that when you breastfeed, it stimulates contractions that collapse your uterus and flatten your stomach. I would lie in bed with Grayson on my nipple and feel my stomach shrinking with each suckle. It felt like I was being eaten from the inside out. And it was painful because of my incision. I caught myself moaning softly as he nursed—I had to power through it and keep hydrating.

Every time I looked in the mirror, my body was smaller, shrinking with every passing day. And I was ravenous. I was sugar-free for my entire pregnancy, with absolutely zero cravings, but all that changed. I ate a whole cheesecake in *three days. And I fantasized about French dips and fried anything. I desperately wanted calories, as many as I could cram in my mouth at once. There were times, between feedings, when I stumbled into the kitchen feeling like a castaway, like I was going to die if I didn't eat something. All I wanted was fat, protein, and carbs.*

Less than a month after giving birth, I'd lost all my baby weight, plus another seventeen pounds. I can eat anything I want without consequence. Calorie counting doesn't even enter my mind. This is the thinnest I've been in my entire life and it's kind of a weird feeling.

I was always a curvy girl with an athletic body and smallish breasts. Now I have big, swollen breasts, thin pins, a little ass, and a perfectly flat stomach. Most of my muscle is gone. When I try to lift something, it's an effort. This experience has made me understand body dysmorphia. I stare in the mirror just blinking, waiting for something to look familiar, because this isn't my body.

But here's the real mindfuck. This is the first time I've used my body for me, to incubate a new life to love and nurture. This isn't about anyone else. This isn't about appealing to the male gaze. This isn't about being fashionable. However, becoming a mother has transformed my body into the ideal. Everyone keeps on telling me how great I look. When you lose seventeen pounds and go up two cup sizes, people sing your praises.

Someone asked if we'd adopted, because I didn't look like I had a baby less than two months ago—sigh. And I've never had so many people ogle my breasts. I'm not sure whether milk-filled breasts press some biological button in people's heads, but they can't keep their eyes off them, male or female. When I answer the door for a delivery, my son cradled in my arms, they still stare like hungry wolves.

Pre-pregnancy, I would have loved the attention. I'd been programmed to seek male attention and inspire female envy (we all are). But now it's kind of creepy and demeaning. I'm the mother of a newborn. There are bigger things on my mind. I don't want to be your fantasy. I don't care if I look sexy. Your compliments ring hollow, because this isn't about you.

It didn't make a difference how long it took to lose the baby weight. That's how things change when you become a parent. You have no time for shallow pursuits. Your focus is on this new little soul—who he'll become and how to best parent him. I daydream about taking him to FAO Schwarz, about the talks we'll have, about our first Easter egg hunt and whom he'll choose to love. For the first time in my life, pleasing others means nothing.

And I remember the exact moment when everything changed. I was sitting in my hospital bed the morning after giving birth when they brought Grayson in for his feeding. It was really our first meeting, because I was too sick and groggy after my C-section for anything to register. They laid him in my arms, and when I looked down into his eyes, time just stopped. In an instant, it all melted away—every anxiety, every insecurity, my need for acceptance. My whole life shifted. I no longer need anyone else to love me. I only need to love this little boy.

Motherhood has been my healing. It has reaffirmed my ideals, my goals, my purpose. I feel that I'm moving into one of the most prolific periods of my life. Everything seems lighter and clearer at the same time. Things move with ease despite the sleepless nights. I know it is going to be a long journey, but with each passing day, I'm becoming a *better person—rising to every challenge, blessed by every moment.*

Who would have thought that at forty-one I'd be enjoying motherhood in size 10 jeans?

7

Self-Care during Parenthood (plus Exercises)

RADICAL SELF-CARE IS an art form. It's not easy. We live in a world that pushes us to work and consume and not spend a lot of time nourishing ourselves and being present. Our society pushes forward this idea of mothers needing to sacrifice all of who they are, their pleasure and needs, to care for another person. And although our responsibilities and our lives shift in a tremendous way when we become mothers, our sexuality, our pleasure, and our identities as individuals are not simply hacked away from us the moment we give birth.

Being still, truly being present with ourselves, and nourishing our bodies, our souls, and our sexual needs and desires is often considered indulgent and discouraged. Well, not here! Radical self-care is transgressive. It's a way that we can change both our emotional outlook on the world and the way we engage with and interact with it. If we are able to transform the way we care for ourselves, we can transform our relationships with our partners, our families, our children, our friends, our neighbors, and the earth.

In this chapter we will talk about radical self-care and how to identify and meet our needs. A helpful mantra that I repeated over and over to my child (and to myself) was "Be gentle to yourself. Be gentle to others. Be gentle to the world around you." Radical self-care is about being gentle to yourself. When we are gentle to ourselves, it enables us to be gentle to others and to the world around us. Our vessel becomes full and overflows with radical love. Transformative love.

Being gentle to ourselves involves cultivating a love for our bodies as they are, and setting gentle, flexible expectations for ourselves. Leaning into what feels good, rather than what is expected of us, and being honest with people about that. Perfecting the art of declining social engagements, or only committing to social engagements that you know will nourish you rather than deplete you.

As we go forward, let's remember to be gentle with ourselves and with each other. The heavy weight of judgments and expectations from those around us during the transition into motherhood can be daunting and oppressive to our spirits and our sexual nature. Let's hold space for one another to be soft-bodied and vulnerable. To talk about our feelings and struggles and our moments of triumph and elation. Let's hold one another up and support one another through this transition and embrace one another in a non-judgmental, open-minded manner as we actively listen.

How to Be an Active Listener for Other Mamas

As moms, we are often given way too much unsolicited advice and not a lot of room to just be as we are. Try to listen to your mama friends as they are talking without interrupting or trying to provide solutions to their problems. Sometimes we just need to talk through things. Be present as someone is speaking and honor her experience as she is speaking it. Often, when we are given space to talk things out, we are able to find our own solutions. You can also try asking questions, like "How did that feel?" "What did that bring up for you?" "What do you need right now in this moment?" "How can we meet that need?" Share these skills with your friends and your partner as helpful guidelines to encouraging active listening.

Make an Agreement to Love Yourself

Ask yourself the following questions and meditate on the answers:

1. What is something you can do each day to engage in self-care?
2. What is something you can do each week to engage in self-care?

An agreement—committing to something in writing—is a clear communication tool and a way to articulate your needs and proactively create change in your life. In making an agreement, like the one below, to radically love yourself, I highly encourage you to have your partner or a close friend sign as a witness. You could also hold witness for a friend's agreement to radical self-care and help one another to stay accountable.

Here are the steps for writing an agreement to radical self-care.

1. State your needs and desires for nourishing your body, sexual self, spirit, and mind.
2. List the radical self-care actions that you would like to commit to, and state how long you will commit to them (a week? a month?).
3. Explore how this radical self-care will manifest in your everyday life.

For example: *Once a month I will get a massage and soak in a hot tub with my friends. Twice a month I will go to an Ecstatic Dance happening with my friends. At least twice a week I will place a note of love and gratitude in my partner's mailbox. I will soak in the tub and eat dinner out under the stars every Thursday night from 7:00 to 9:00 p.m. This will be my sacred renewal time in which I can meditate and care for myself.*

Treat this document as a working agreement and refer back to it on a monthly basis. If something isn't working, find out why and change it. Maybe you need more resources or more help in order to meet the radical self-care needs that you have. Maybe your radical self-care has to be temporarily modified to fit into your current new mama life. This agreement should be used as a communication tool. If it feels obligatory, then it needs to change. Leave room for change and acknowledge that change is okay. That what you desire will change. And that there are no rules for what your relationship or your expression of radical self-care has to look like. Set an expiration date for review and revision.

Intimacy Exercise: Three Needs, Three Gifts

This is an exercise that was first presented to me by my therapist, and it was so very helpful in my own relationship that I now incorporate it into my sex and relationship workshop curriculum. I generally do this exercise with my partner at our weekly household meeting as we examine our upcoming week and reflect on the past week and what our current needs and gifts may be.

This is an exercise I especially like to do during difficult weeks, or weeks when I know that either my partner or I will need a little extra support. It aids in articulating what your needs are and how you would like them met. Both you and your partner should write down three things that you need from your partner that week, and three things that you can offer to your partner to help your partner through the week emotionally or physically. This might look something like:

Partner I:

Needs:
1. Intimacy and connection with my partner
2. Time with my friends to go dancing
3. To work out at the gym or go jogging

What I can give:
1. Foot massage
2. Cooking dinner (maybe we can find a fun way to do the dishes after the little one is asleep—kitchen sex?)
3. Taking the baby for a stroll on Saturday morning so you can sleep in

Partner 2:
Needs:
1. Sleep and relaxation
2. Intimacy with my partner without the baby around
3. A sense of home and security—a home-cooked meal would be great

What I can give:
1. Hiring a sitter for one night
2. Date night: Dinner out, then hotel sex or parking in the car like teenagers
3. Going in to work late on Friday so you can go jogging

What do your and your partner's needs and gifts look like? Are your partner's needs different from what you expected? Post this list where you can see it throughout the week and take care of any logistics, such as booking a sitter or sorting out which day you will cook dinner. Pre-planning alleviates stress and creates a sense of stability. Stress is counterproductive to nurturing our libidos. Eliminate stress, increase communication, support one another in your needs, and watch the love and connection pour in.

Visualization Exercise

This exercise requires your eyes to be closed, so use a recording device or the voice memo function on your phone to record the following paragraphs so that you both can listen to it while you experience the exercise. Speak slowly, clearly, and audibly so that you are not struggling to make out the words.

Lie down on the ground, beside your partner but not touching. Close your eyes. Have your palms facing upward toward the ceiling. Slowly allow your body to settle and become heavy against the earth. If there is any tension in your body, release it. We are releasing tension and welcoming warmth and love and erotic energy into our bodies. Bring a consciousness to the rise and fall of your breath, and use your breath to release tension. If your shoulders or neck or ankles are holding tension, bring some gentle movement to those areas, one at a time. As you gently rock, circle, or sway that part of your body, let tension fall away with your exhale. Your legs should be hip-width apart. As you breathe, start to bring a consciousness to the space between your legs. With each breath, allow the energy that is radiating between your legs to grow. I like to visualize a ball of energy—a tiny sun between my legs. Give it a color—pink, orange, gold, red—a warm ball of energy pulsating and growing, its light growing in intensity with each breath. On your deep inhale, tighten your PC muscles and tilt your pelvis downward. On your exhale, release your PC muscles, pushing outward and tilting your pelvis up. Allow your pelvis to circle and sway, building energy with your breath and allowing your ball of energy to grow bigger. The sun-like warmth and energy is growing, and the ball's rays are shooting off from its center. Warm light encircles your core, your abdomen, your spine, finding its way up your chest, encircling your heart and reaching out to your extremities—your arms, your legs, your fingers, your toes, all tingling. As this light and energy beams from your toes and your fingers, allow your exhale to release with texture. Deep belly moans and growls, howls and earthy calls of the wild. Let your animal spirit exhale whatever sounds rest deep between your legs, from your cunt, your cock, your gut, your womb. Arch your back as you call out to the earth, a collective cry that swoops up the orgasmic energy of every ecstatic creature that has fucked before you. Allow that energy to churn deep inside you as you pulse and rock your pelvis, never forgetting your radiant beauty, your power, your pleasure, and your breath.

Breathe this energy, this ecstasy, out in a gift to yourself and to your partner. Imagine your erotic energy taking hold of your partner and drawing your partner close to your body. Slowly, with great power and intention, reach out your hand and lightly touch your partner. Experience the great intensity of the smallest touch with the greatest energy. Allow your hand to explore your partner's hand as you continue with your breath, with the movement of your pelvis, the movement of energy through your body. Allow your hand to make love to your partner's hand, discovering its ultimate sensuality in touch. Align your breath with that of your partner and let your hand find its way atop your partner's chest. You can stay in this moment in ecstatic breath and energy with your partner, or feel free to allow this exercise to act as a catalyst for more physical sexual play—oral sex, intercourse, or any other intimacy that might feel inspiring in this moment as you slowly, with breath and intention, gift one another with the radical pleasure that you have both cultivated for one another.

TRANSITIONS INTO MOTHERHOOD
WITH NATASHIA FUKSMAN, MA

Transitions are so overwhelming, and what can add to that is that when you're in a new phase in your life, you don't necessarily know what is grounding.

It's going to be a process to find out what is helpful or supportive for you at this stage. There are three things that really stand out to me, and that are not encouraged enough throughout this transitional period—firstly, individual reflective time. Secondly, some reflective couple time, even if it's just once a week in the beginning. New parents are undergoing a massive change of focus, and they will need time and space to figure out how to meet each other again now that they've both developed new relationships that are just as important as the relationship they have made with one another. They need time to figure themselves out as a couple again now that they have this new addition in their lives. Thirdly, extended community time that includes other women who are in or around the same stage of motherhood and make the woman feel safe to explore what is safe for her in this time of transition.

A SEXY MAMA'S POV
WITH SEXPERT JAMYE WAXMAN, M.ED.

You might not want sex when you're pregnant. I know—shocker, right?

The real problem is that you might feel bad about not wanting sex during pregnancy, especially when so many people are telling you just how good pregnant sex can be. You'll hear that it's the best, juiciest sex you'll never get to have again (hell, yes!). You'll hear that now that you have as many hormones as a pubescent boy (or at least that is how it feels at times), and that you'll want to do the humpty dance all day long. And you'll be advised to get it on in positions that make you feel confident that you won't hurt the fetus. That's all great information, but sometimes that won't make you feel great.

You may feel even worse when it's your partner who doesn't want sex because he or she is going through his or her own changes, and dealing with excitement, anxiety, and stress too. These feelings can lead to a lot of not feeling, and that not feeling can lead to a lot more of the things you don't want to feel when you're pregnant. And while I managed to stay positive during my pregnancy, I was positively not as sexual as I thought I would be.

When you're a sex educator, like I am, it's a real challenge to be okay with not having sex, and to tell others it's okay not to have sex. At first I was so focused on exploring my sexuality and wanting to have the best pregnant sex I could have that when I wasn't having sex, I felt like I was doing this pregnancy wrong. Later, I got down on myself for not wanting sex. I got down on my partner for not wanting sex. I got down on the notion that women who have orgasmic births are doing it better, and I began feeling sad about the fact that I wasn't having much of an orgasmic pre-birth either.

While my girlfriends were glowing about how great pregnant sex was for them, I began harboring this fear that not only was I not carpe diem-ing the fuck out of the pregnancy, I was failing at my job and at this experience. But when my daughter was lying so low that I thought my vagina was going to fall out between my legs, I didn't want sex. When my acid reflux was burning though my mouth, I didn't want sex. When it felt like a thousand bees were stinging my boobs every time I walked through the freezer aisle at the grocery store, I didn't want sex. And when I peed a little on the supermarket floor after a big sneeze, I didn't feel sexy—I felt leaky. And then I got over myself.

You may feel bad about having too little sex because you think you should want sex. Or maybe you think your partner should want to bask in the glow of your bodacious pregnant belly. Popular magazines have you believe that these things are fact—that every partner wants his or her baby mama more when she's with child. That's just not true—not always.

At times when I did want sex, but my partner's and my sex drives didn't sync, I had orgasms with my trusty Eroscillator. It wasn't as pretty or as warm as my partner, but I am a believer in keeping the vag pumped up and the blood flowing, and I love masturbation (heck, I wrote a book on it). I enjoyed every single solo moment I could muster, and in the end, when my water broke, I was doing this very thing that I love.

What I ultimately learned was that there is no one way that your sexuality will play out when you're pregnant.

And the only thing about sex and pregnancy that I can say with any degree of certainty is that your body will change, and so will your desires, needs, and wants. And whether you have lots of sex, or just a little, the more you can love yourself through the experience, the more you can love (and laugh at) yourself during pregnancy.

8

Mantras, Affirmations, Meditation, Yoga

CHANGE **AND** *LOSS* **CAN** be terrifying words, yet every day that we continue our life journey we are changing, evolving, experiencing loss and gaining new perspectives. Life is not static, and this becomes radically apparent as we begin our journey into motherhood. Our bodies, our needs, our desires, our views of life expand and change. This doesn't mean cashing in your sexy lingerie for sleep deprivation and chapped nipples, but it does mean that your perspective on life and your role in life are transforming and evolving, and so is your body.

Hormonally you are in overdrive, and physically there are buckets full of changes that you can expect, internally and externally, throughout pregnancy, including swollen ankles, fluid retention, weight gain, stretch marks, and engorged breasts. Postpartum, you can expect hair loss, leaky breasts, more stretch marks, and a body that just spent nine months creating a baby and morphing like crazy to do so.

Through these challenging transitions you might experience a loss of identity, a loss of confidence, or even depression. It can be difficult to be in a body that doesn't feel like it fits, and once you are in full-on mama mode, there's no time to recalibrate, because your every waking hour is devoted to the surviving and thriving of your offspring. Through these many transitions and emotional roller coasters both before and after entering motherhood, I've found that mindfulness techniques such as mantras, affirmations, meditations, and yoga have been my North Star, my grounding practice that brings me back to solid footing and helps me to journey onward.

In this chapter you will find some techniques that I use and have found useful, explained by some of my fellow sexy mamas: yoga experts Jardana Peacock and Isabelle Boesch and sex educator Eri Kardos.

Mantras

Jardana Peacock is an activist and yoga teacher as well as a mother of two.

Jardana: During my second pregnancy, I enrolled in an advanced tantric yoga training and traveled to India to study yoga. So this was a really exceptional year, compounded by the fact that I was pregnant!

I had a beautiful Sanskrit teacher, Arvind Pare, during my time in India. Arvind gave poetic lectures on the meaning of Vedic texts and ancient mantras. Ganesha is a very popular god in Hinduism (this is the god with the elephant head); however, I had never really related to him. Arvind shared a beautiful story about the god Ganesha who had blue skin that sparkled like a million stars, and my relationship to Ganesha immediately changed—this image was so powerful for me, it brought tears to my eyes. Ganesha is a beautiful, grounding god who both places and removes obstacles in our lives. It is said that Ganesha will not place any obstacle in your path that you are not able to overcome. I began a pretty steady practice in India and afterward of working with Ganesha. My mantra was "Om Ganesha Namah," which means "I bow to Ganesha, I honor Ganesha and what he stands for."

I also began a practice with Chinnamasta during my second pregnancy. Chinnamasta is a fierce warrior goddess who cuts off her own head when her children are hungry and then, with her severed head, feeds herself and her two children. I immediately related to her energy as a nurturer, a warrior, and also a sexually vibrant being. Sexual trauma survivors often find powerful resilience and healing inside of ourselves— Chinnamasta became that reminder for me.

There are specific mantras for the goddesses, but in my practice I found that the energy of the goddesses should be handled with reverence. I do not recommend working with the fierce warrior goddesses (Chinnamasta, Kali, and Durga) without the supervision of a teacher, unless you are an extremely seasoned practitioner. If you are energy-sensitive, as I am, I believe you can harm yourself without supervision. I was under the supervision of a teacher and still at times felt overwhelmed by their energy. My sole mantra has been "Om Ganesha Namah" for over a year, both before and during pregnancy and now as a mama of two. I do meditations with the goddesses, but I'm not ready for more at this point.

My advice for folks wanting to learn more about mantras is to read the book *Awakening Shakti: The Transformative Power of the Goddesses of Yoga*, specifically focusing on Lakshmi, the goddess of abundance, and Saraswati, the goddess of insight, inspiration, and creativity. These goddesses are more grounding, like Ganesha. However, Chinnamasta and Durga are also powerful during pregnancy if handled with care and under a trusted teacher's direction.

Isabelle Boesch has taught yoga to mothers and children for the past ten years.

Isabelle: "This too shall pass." I like this mantra because when I'm going through hell (toddler meltdown, baby who won't nap, husband who just doesn't get it), it reminds me to keep on going toward the light at the end of the tunnel. And when I am in one of those super-yummy mom moments (nursing baby looks up at me with a big drippy smile; toddler says, "Mommy, I put my shoes on all by myself!"; husband does the dishes without me even asking), I really savor it and remember that these moments are precious.

Another mantra that I used very successfully in labor was "YES!" I wasn't saying "Yes" in the sense that I loved every moment, but rather, "Yes, this is happening now." It helped me stay present and ride the waves. Now that I'm a mama of two (four years and two months old) I find myself saying "Yes" again, often! Also, that "Yes" mantra during sex brings me to even higher heights. Not that I've had sex yet since my son was born. And I say "Yes" even to that, because I know that this short sex-free stage in our marriage will pass. I guess what is embedded in that *yes* is a message to myself that I am seen by myself, that I am witnessing my own experience. It makes this path of being a stay-at-home mom a little more bearable and a little less lonely.

If you want to try working with a mantra, I would ask you to close your eyes and think of your first memory. See yourself as a child. What would you say to that child to comfort her? How would she want to be touched? Maybe she wants to hear "I will never leave you" or "You are unconditionally loved" or "That was really hard, and *look,* you got through it. I'm so proud of you." Usually these same words of comfort can be used as mantras, because they are still comforting.

Eri: During my pregnancy, my mantra was "I was born to do this!" I felt so alive during my pregnancy. I felt like Superwoman! Creating new life inspired me to write a book, go on a national speaking tour across eleven states, and hike through eight national parks. It was incredible.

Postpartum, my mantra became "Breathe." I was really lucky to have a huge community of support after giving birth. Even so, I had moments of exhaustion and being overwhelmed. It was such a strange experience to go from carrying this little one around inside of me to having him outside and requiring so much more of me! I had lost much of my sense of self once I was no longer pregnant. I struggled with feelings of loneliness and emptiness. Feeding was harder than I expected, and it was difficult not to have a loud inner critic. I had to be very intentional about being gentle with myself and allowing myself to stay present with whatever emotions arose. Making time to breathe, cry, take hot showers, and be held like a baby by my lover pulled me through this intensely joyous and intensely challenging phase.

Settling into new motherhood, I developed the mantra "Oh my God, I am a MILF!" About three weeks after giving birth I was hungry for sex. I checked in with my body and moved slowly as we engaged in foreplay. All of a sudden it struck me that my partner still found me attractive! Even as a sex-positive educator, I subconsciously carried around toxic stories about how women are no longer attractive once they become moms. This could not be further from the truth. Now I am just more grounded and powerful. I've been delighted to see the types of individuals who are flirting with and pursing me; they are all yummy, powerful people. Also, my boobs have never looked so good!

My tip to women looking to find their mantras in each stage of this journey: Journal, meditate, and read *Birthing from Within* by Ina May. Feel your way into this sacred rite of passage and embrace the goddess warrior that you are. Whatever comes, this is your journey.

Affirmations

Jardana: An affirmation that I have used in motherhood is "I love my life exactly as it is." This affirmation has helped me to be in the moment, to stop trying to "fix" everything or get out of a situation I wish was going differently—whether that's wanting my four-year-old to stop screaming in a store or my fussy baby to go to sleep, or the times when I feel like I don't have enough time to grow my holistic healing business in the ways that I would like. This has also given me permission to stop trying to be a "supermom" and listen to my needs—which, during the postpartum stage, were often to simply rest!

Another affirmation that I love is from the Buddhist meditation teacher Thich Nhat Hanh, and it is "I see you and I love you." This is from his work on love. He states that when you really see who is in front of you, you drop yourself into that person's presence. I use this with my partner when we are arguing, and it helps me hear him and appreciate him more. I use this with my child and with my baby to drop into the moment with them in bigger ways.

When it comes time to determine an affirmation, I lead my clients in a process that looks something like this:

Answer these questions.

What are your fears [around this pregnancy/parenthood]?

How do you want to feel in this moment [during pregnancy, labor, parenthood]?

Describe yourself as a superhero. What do you wear? How do you act? What is your greatest power?

Now circle words that sparkle for you, that stir you. Create an affirmation based on these words.

For example:

I am radiant.

I am a warrior.

My baby and I are working together in magical tandem.

Isabelle: My favorite affirmation is "It is not anyone else's job to approve of/like/love me/my choices/my body." That is my job, and it's a very important job.

I respect my children and myself by welcoming all feelings to show up. My mothering body is beautiful. I can't do it all. I make wise choices and do one thing at a time.

I often get caught up in worrying what others will think of me. In early motherhood, I bought as many parenting books as I could get my hands on and read them all. The conflicting advice drove me crazy because I wanted to do the "right thing." Now, the second time around, I'm learning (and affirming) that I am the expert and that others' opinions of me are theirs and I can't do anything to change them. By pinpointing an area that was giving me trouble, I could then ask myself what thoughts go through my head when I experience negative emotions. For instance, one thought I often had was "I should be doing more with my day." This is a painful thought because I am just not *able* to do the things I used to be able to do now that I am caring for an infant twenty-four seven. It sets me up for failure. So I ask myself, "Is this true? *Should* I be doing more?" The answer came quickly: "NO!" And so my affirmation became, "I shouldn't do more. I am doing enough."

Meditation

Jardana: During pregnancy, I practiced a really lovely meditation called the ocean/fire meditation. I first started with a four-part breathing practice, breathing into my lower abdomen, belly, heart, and throat and then repeating that cycle a few times. Then I focused on my heart area and imagined that there was an ocean in my heart. Every thought or distraction that entered into my mind, I would feed it to the ocean and let it dissolve. This is a very grounding meditation and has a similar effect to yoga nidra (explained later in this chapter). It leads you deeper into the parasympathetic nervous system and helps create a lot of spaciousness and peace inside the body. This is a perfect meditation to manage the anxiety, fear, anticipation, joy, and even trauma that surfaces during pregnancy, labor, and parenting.

During birth, I used a powerful meditation with the goddess Durga, who is the goddess of justice, protection, and inner strength. She is also the power behind spiritual awakening and kundalini energy. I invoked Durga the day I gave birth and experienced a deeply sexual and spiritual birthing experience.

According to myth, Durga is the goddess who saved the world, but only when she was asked. My partner and I meditated the morning of August 3. We imagined Durga riding with us on her lion and through us. We asked Durga for protection during the birth. Later that day, my labor began.

Toward the end of my labor, a large contraction came over me like a wave, and my body took over. Everything disappeared. I imagined Durga inside of me. She rode a golden lion. I imagined golden light streaming into my body and rooting me to the core of the earth. I imagined that I was glistening radiant golden light. I felt powerful, fierce, beautiful, and full of sexual energy. My voice moaned deep as I squatted. The world around me disappeared. For about thirty minutes, I became one with my body, empowered in my labor and deeply connected to my babe.

August Elwyn came into the world with ease. I was on all fours and the midwife slid him underneath me. It felt like complete magic. My relief and joy, and the deep presence I experienced, were sacred. I scooped him into my arms and held him for the next hour as his umbilical cord pulsed. This moment felt enlightened. I felt held and connected to my community, family, and spirituality. I became Durga in that hospital room, and my beautiful baby lit up the night with pure love.

Isabelle: I really like guided meditations and have been using an app on my phone called Headspace for a while. I like that it tracks how often I use it, and the meditations are different each day. I feel like I get credit for each time I meditate, which works really well for me. So not only do I get the benefit of crossing something off of my to-do list first thing in the morning (which is when I meditate—before the rest of the family wakes up), but I also get the benefit of clearing my mind and starting fresh. The days I don't meditate, I feel noticeably off.

I find motherhood to be a restless time. My mind has a hard time letting go of thoughts and thinking. It believes that it always has to be working. I, on the other hand, know that it doesn't, that it's okay to relax. This is why a guided meditation works so well for moms—because it reminds us to come back to our focus.

Eri: My partner invited me into this exercise. I encourage you to start your day off with it. I placed my hands on my belly to do this while pregnant. If a partner was with me, he or she would stand behind me and wrap their arms around me to touch my belly and breathe with me.

Five Breaths Meditation:

1. Stand with your feet hip-width apart, or sit in the lotus position.
2. Close your eyes.
3. With the first inhale and exhale, practice smiling.
4. With the second inhale and exhale, fill yourself with gratitude.
5. With the third inhale and exhale, forgive others.
6. With the fourth inhale and exhale, forgive yourself.
7. With the fifth inhale and exhale, set your intention for the day.

Yoga

Jardana: During my pregnancy, I was involved in a forty-day practice right before birth. Part of that practice involved yoga nidra, which is a deeply relaxing form of yoga. *Yoga nidra* means "deep sleep." You actually don't move at all, but instead dive into the emotional, mental, and spiritual body by following a set of instructions. I recommend Rolf Sovik's explanation, found on Yoga International's website (https://yogainternational.com/). You can also find recordings online or make your own by recording yourself reading the instructions. Yoga nidra should be practiced for at least thirty minutes. This form of yoga nourishes your body and prepares it for labor. During my first pregnancy, my practice was very different. I practiced traditional Ashtanga yoga, which is a more difficult physical practice. My entry into parenthood with my first child was extremely challenging, and it took me a long time to connect to my child—some of which was related to unprocessed trauma that surfaced during labor. However, I believe part of it also had to do with my yoga practice. My recent postpartum period with my second child was full of a lot of joy and ease. The transition from pregnancy to parenting two little ones was graceful. Prior to birth, I was working with my body instead of pushing it. Yoga nidra restored my body and filled it with the energy it needed to labor. The nidra practice was also a radical act of self-care. I am a very motivated and inspired woman; it's hard for me to slow down. However, yoga nidra allowed me the opportunity to be with my growing baby and myself during pregnancy and after birth in a deeply intimate way.

I started practicing hot yoga after giving birth. My body felt so tired and tense postpartum. Vinyasa was too hard on me. I wanted to move a little more than with yoga nidra, although I still practiced it at least once a week. Hot yoga made me feel strong and detoxed my body in ways that felt right. Oftentimes I would only participate in the asana poses for about thirty minutes and then lie in final rest for the remaining class time. My body still needed rest, but it also needed movement.

My offering around finding what is right for you is this: Find a balance between a strength-based practice and a resting practice. Your body needs both. Don't push yourself physically until at least six months after delivery. Even now, I lie down when in yoga class when I start to feel tired. I also try to only give fifty to sixty percent effort to the poses. Some days I give more and some days less. I remind myself, "My practice is perfect as it is. My body is beautiful as it is."

My practice outside of a class setting involves lighting a candle at my altar and practicing yoga nidra or a slow asana that really focuses on strengthening my pelvic floor and gets deep into my hips. I also practice holding warrior poses for up to three minutes. A great way to listen to what your body and mind need is to blindfold yourself, or, if that feels uncomfortable, close your eyes and move only when you feel the desire. This helps you get out of your mind and into your body. I also spend time breathing (pranayama) and meditating.

During pregnancy and immediately afterward, the body taps into a place of deep intuition and power. Tap into this truth and the power within. Remember, you are already perfect, and you have all the answers you need inside. You are going to rock it, beautiful!

Isabelle: *Any* form of self-care is going to enliven your life as a mother. One of the simplest poses (although not the easiest) is tadasana. It is the foundational posture for all standing poses. The idea is to learn correct alignment, muscle movements, and mindset so that poses you do in the future have the same integrity. As a mom, I often have a crooked stance from holding my child on one hip, or rounded shoulders from crooning at or nursing my baby. Tadasana encourages me to stand up tall, stacking my bones. If I want to see what good alignment looks like, I need look no further than my own daughter. She stands tall (when she stands still, which is rarely), and she allows for the natural curves of her spine.

The strength and empowerment of motherhood, while powerful, are also soft and supple. Early motherhood is a time of many changes, when a woman has to adapt to life with a baby. It can be a challenging time that many of us are not prepared for. One of the biggest shockers for me was the lack of time I had for myself. Before I had children, I luxuriated in my yoga practice. Being a caregiver for a tiny little being twenty-four seven is a big responsibility. Those early weeks and months are often a time of insecurity for moms. It is extremely important for them to take care of themselves so that they can care for their little ones. One of the hardest things for me was when my baby would cry for no apparent reason. It was during these times that my yoga practice really served me. I wasn't doing poses per se, but I found myself breathing deeply and even chanting "om." It centers and calms me, and it soothes my baby too. Deep ujjayi breathing combined with walking or rocking is good medicine.

I experienced postpartum depression with my first daughter, and a regular yoga practice really helped me, as did yoga philosophy. It reminded me to be a witness to my emotions.

Finally, another aspect that we can think about and cultivate is bhakti yoga, or devotional yoga. As mothers, we are practicing the ultimate bhakti yoga. Motherhood is an act of complete devotion; we can call it devotional yoga. So even if we do not have time to practice asanas and pranayama, we can try to cultivate this devotional aspect throughout the day (and night!). Learn to adjust and be flexible, leaving our expectations for ourselves and even for our babies behind. Karma yoga is another form of yoga we can do; as mothers, we have to be selfless, and one of our duties is to look after, nurture, and love our child in the best possible way, leaving aside expectations. This is our dharma. Practicing yoga in this way is the ultimate yoga, and in this way we can cultivate that divine female energy that allowed us to create the wonderful baby we have in our lives.

9

Fitness after Baby

WHEN WE TAKE CARE of our bodies and get our bodies moving, everything improves. Our mood, our physical health and strength, our circulation, and our libido. Just because you become pregnant doesn't mean that your physical activity needs to stop. There were definitely points during my pregnancy at which I felt totally exhausted and all I needed was to sleep. But moving my body kept me feeling strong, inspired, and super sexy.

I'm an urban mama, and during my pregnancy I was living in San Francisco in the Haight neighborhood. If you are unfamiliar with San Francisco, it is one very hilly city. I haven't driven in years since I moved to the Bay Area, and I walk everywhere. This didn't stop when I became pregnant. I kept on walking, everywhere, even up those huge hills in the Haight. In fact, that's how I got my labor moving—hiking hills in San Francisco and eating super-spicy burritos! I also kept working out, although I greatly modified my workouts. Your body changes during pregnancy.

Once I got into my second trimester, I stopped doing aerial performance. I kept walking, biking, and swimming, as well as dancing and doing yoga. Yoga was possibly the most helpful of all the physical exercises that I engaged in during pregnancy. It helped me to relax and feel bonded to the other women in my class. I didn't feel so alone, and slowly I started to build community with other soon-to-be moms who were invested in their wellness. When I was no longer able to do much else and was as round as a beach ball in my third trimester, yoga kept me centered and feeling good about my body. It helped me to continue feeling connected to my sexuality, and to honor the vessel that housed my child as well as the person I was and the person I was becoming.

Whether it's yoga, dancing, or daily walks, find ways to move your body and stay active (unless otherwise advised by your doctor).

After baby arrived, I remember walking to the Gold's Gym in the Castro to sign up for a membership with my baby in tow. Hot gay men abounded, pumping iron and running laps, and here I was, the stretched-out, soft and curvy postpartum mom with leaky breasts and a screaming child strolling into the gym. I believe I was the only woman there, and definitely the only mom. But I knew I needed to get active again. I needed to get back on the treadmill. I needed to get moving. I signed up for a membership as I pulled out my breast and nursed my crying child in the lobby. I did find my way back to the gym and got moving on the treadmill and cardio machines. And it felt good. It felt good to be dripping in sweat and racing toward a different version of myself, Le Tigre blaring in my headphones as I jogged. My milky breasts would still squirt and leak and I'd sometimes have to leave early or have the sitter just stroll around the neighborhood with my baby while I worked out. But I found ways to make it work.

Being active made me feel like myself. It gave me the gift of time that was mine—even if it was a quick twenty-minute jog. It recharged me for the rest of the day and gave me energy on days when I was exhausted from sleepless nights. When I stepped back on the treadmill and started jogging and even lifting weights, it was obvious that my body strength was very different from what it was pre-baby. My muscles were weak. I was used to being so strong. To being able to exhaust my muscles—but wow, doing a sit-up after birthing a baby was hard, and Kegels (flexing of the PC muscles) were difficult! Really, it was so hard. My brain was telling my muscles what to do, but they were so weak. It was frustrating to know that the things I'd been able to do before were now so difficult. And it was frustrating to wonder, *Will these activities be difficult forever?* They weren't. And I kept at it. It took almost a year before I was able to get my core strength back to a point where I could do the kind of aerial performance that I was used to doing pre-baby. And that first time I was back in the air, it was magic. It felt so radically empowering. The hip and pelvic area really open and loosen their ligaments in the third trimester, and it took a while to strengthen those ligaments and muscles post-baby before I could engage in aerial performance and suspensions. But I got there.

I kept moving, and it helped. I felt like I was going somewhere, and that slowly I was becoming stronger and very slowly reclaiming my body that was slowly healing and finding its own strength once again.

A SEXY MAMA'S POV
WITH YOGA EXPERT, SURFER, GYMNAST, AND MASSAGE THERAPIST CARA KELSEY

During pregnancy I really had to tell myself that it was okay not to feel sexy. My sexuality is part of my identity, and not feeling connected to that was really hard for me. I had to remind myself that I was more than a sexual being and that I would find and fall in love with a new part of me that I didn't have room to discover before.

I reminded myself that I was making a human; I was a creator. That made me feel powerful. It made all the struggles that I faced during my pregnancy worth it. Everything is temporary is a mantra I used and still use. It puts things into perspective for me. My body has gone through many different things and looked many different ways and I have always learned to love it. The same can be said about my sense of self; my sexuality was not always empowering to me, but I taught myself how to love my sexuality. I have struggled and triumphed and will continue to do so. Self-love is loving the parts of yourself you don't like.

That mantra reminded me to be gentle with myself. It still reminds me to treat myself the way I want my daughter to treat herself and to talk to myself the way I want her to talk to herself.

Taking time to breathe and be in my body has always been the baseline of my meditation. Adding mantras in the morning helps me set up my self-talk for the day, and doing a yoga sequence or stretch routine helps me feel in my body and listen to what it needs. Learning to be still with a baby attached to me—or, now, with a toddler attached to me—has been a challenge. Meditation looks different now. Sometimes it's me and my child dancing and taking loud breaths, sometimes it's me counting my breaths and focusing on my heart with my child crawling all over me, but it helps.

Over the past three years I have done a lot of meditation focused on being in my body and feeling sexual again. I sat at night and focused my breath toward my root chakra. I would rock my pelvis while breathing to move more energy and bring more of my focus to my vulva and my whole pelvis. I would take time in the shower or during my daughter's nap to masturbate, not to get off, necessarily, but to consciously reconnect with my body. Just recently my partner and I started meditating together, and during some meditations we felt each other breathe and took turns breathing in and out.

I make sure that I am getting some form of regular massage, which I think can be a form of meditation. I believe that receiving touch on a regular basis helps me stay in tune with what my body needs, lets me feel *nurtured and cared for, reduces my stress and anxiety, and makes it easier for me to touch other people.*

The more comfortable I get with nonsexual touch and being in my body, the more I am able to be in my body during sexual expression. Meditation is a practice and looks different for everyone. Most importantly I believe in playing with meditation. Don't be hard on yourself. Give yourself the space to work it out, even if that looks like counting breaths while you take a hot shower or dancing in your living room to get energy or anxiety out. Meditation is a tool, and it should not be a source of stress.

I came up with a mini yoga sequence that I can do every day. I combined four or five poses into a flow and try to do it every morning. It can take less than five minutes, depending on how many times I repeat the sequence. The more I repeat it, the more it becomes a moving meditation. I use cat-cow, downward-facing dog, plank, cobra, and child's pose as my flow. Other poses I like are eagle and bound angle. When I was younger, I struggled a lot with my period. I had horrible cramps that made me vomit and horrible PMS. I decided to be proactive and looked up diet tips and yoga poses that could help. I ended up making flash cards with pictures of the poses and notes on their benefits. That way, I could put the flash cards together in different ways to make different sequences. This made yoga accessible for me; I could lay the flash cards on the floor or memorize them. I still have those flash cards. I did the same thing with this mini sequence. Since we have the Internet now, I just Googled "yoga for sexual desire" and selected the poses that resonated with me. All the poses I chose focus on drawing awareness to your body through chest or hip openers, or contracting and drawing energy in, then releasing the contraction. My partner mentioned that he wanted to watch me do my sequence naked. I was very insecure about the idea at first, but now I highly recommend that everyone try naked yoga by themselves or with a partner. It has become another way to make my self-care sexy and for me to become even more comfortable in my body and being naked.

10

Family Management Tips and Tricks

"MOMMY IS GOING TO take some mommy time for a few minutes." This is a phrase that I say to my child when I need a break or a breather. If I don't listen to my body and take the time and space I need, I end up really regretting it. Sometimes mommy just needs to eat. Sometimes I need to take a five-minute breather on the porch before I deal with the room that is now covered in finger paint. Sometimes it's preemptive, and I'm thinking ahead about what my needs are based on our schedule. Sometimes life happens, and I need to ask for small chunks of mommy time to deal with everyday stresses that come up with work, deadlines, and family issues. Sometimes mothering doesn't leave a lot of space for your own emotions and needs, and you have to advocate for that space and time in a way that your children can understand while still letting them know they are loved and safe and cared for.

One of my favorite ways to reset and find space for my own emotional well-being is by either getting a sitter or a friend to watch my child while I take time to journal in a park, or, if I have my child with me, taking a "wellness day" and going to the beach or out to the redwoods. Being out in nature with my feet in the soil or the sand helps me to breathe more deeply and feel connected to the earth and to life. I'm able to breathe a little more deeply when I'm out in nature, and so is my child. My little one is an emotional barometer. If I'm upset or distressed about something, it affects not only me but my child. Taking care of myself and my own emotional well-being is taking care of my child's emotional well-being.

Through parenting, I've discovered tools that help us to process our emotions and talk about our feelings when life feels a bit overwhelming. In the same way that I advocate for parents to breathe to move energy around, our children can learn to breathe to let go of tension in their body too. One tool I use with my child is called birthday breaths.

Birthday Breaths

Put up your five fingers about twelve inches from your child's face and ask him or her to blow out the candles. Upon his or her first deep belly breath, put one of your fingers down, signifying that your child blew out the candle. Upon the second deep belly breath, put another finger down, signifying blowing out the second candle. Continue this until your child has blown out all five "candles."

When I'm feeling tense or experiencing big emotions, my four-year-old returns the favor and says "Birthday breaths, mom." and puts up five fingers for me so that I can practice my own breathing.

Coloring

Coloring is a calming, meditative practice not only for children but also for grown-ups. Get your own coloring book to use and color with your child. Decide beforehand whether or not your coloring book and crayons are a sharing item. It's okay to have your own things that are not for your child. It's important to have both space and objects of our own. And it's okay for your child to have special things that are not for sharing either. Not everything has to be shared.

Now that my child is four years old, they don't nap, but they still need daily "decompression" from their day at preschool. At 2:00 p.m. every day, we lower the lights, put on the "twinkle lights," put on some calming music, and do quiet activities like coloring. If my child doesn't get this chill self-care time, it's radically noticeable. They need to get a break from the high level of stimulus that they have experienced at school and refill their vessel, and I do too.

If mommy's vessel is empty, everyone suffers. Don't let everyone—including yourself—suffer. Make mommy time a necessity and work regular self-care into the schedule.

Naughty Time

Sometimes mommy time means that mommy and her partner need alone time together to be intimate. Sometimes it means that mommy needs mommy time to be intimate with herself. Finding time to engage in intimacy is critical to our well-being. It's absolutely possible as a mom, but it takes creative thinking and boundaries. Just remember: Every time you stick up for your own needs and boundaries, you are modeling and teaching your child how to ask for the space, privacy, and things that they need.

One of my favorite times to masturbate was nap time, but now my child has grown out of naps. But I still enjoy an early-evening masturbation session after my little one is in bed and before my husband is home from work. The shower can also be a great place either to pleasure yourself or for you and your partner to find space and time for sex. A handheld shower nozzle can provide orgasmic clitoral stimulation, as can many of the waterproof sex toys that can live on the top shelf of your shower. Our little one also knows that on the weekends they can watch morning cartoons while mommy and daddy have alone time. They understand that this is a time when we want space and privacy. We have empowered them with language to ask for the space and privacy that they need too.

Come Together: Connecting with Other Moms

Sometimes mommy time means we need some time with other moms who understand what we are going through. We need support so that we don't feel alone. Sometimes it can feel like our early days of motherhood are spent in a breastfeeding oxytocin haze of naps and dirty diapers and sleep deprivation. We're quarantined in a service-oriented relationship to our nonverbal children. Sometimes we just need to be around other adults who get it and who are nonjudgmental and empathetic because they are going through the same thing.

About a month after the birth of my daughter, I started a mom's group called the Sexy Mamas Social Club. I wanted to find a group of women who understood me and accepted me for the mom that I was. I wanted a group of women who were interested in sex and talking about sex and how pregnancy and motherhood had affected their sex lives and how they were adjusting. A place where we could support one another and inspire and encourage one another. It was a truly supportive group of sex-positive mamas that came together. There were sex educators, kinksters, poly folk, sex workers, queers, and sex radicals who had all chosen to become parents and were learning the ropes as we went along. We learned from one another and shared resources, and I'm still good friends with many of the Sexy Mamas today. Some of them even contributed to this book!

I highly recommend reaching out and finding a group of women who you feel comfortable talking with. If you can't find a sex-positive mom's group, start a Sexy Mamas Social Club of your very own in your own city. Just pick a place, date, and time; send out the invites; and post on social media. There are also online resources like Meetup, which can be a good place to post about groups or to find an already existing group.

It's a Process

Sometimes our minds can become so clouded with emotion that it is difficult to sort out the actual problem and pinpoint the change that we need to make in order to manifest the support and care that we need. Purging everything that's clouding your mind and getting it out on paper in an uncensored writing exercise can give you space to just let it all out. Dig into the layers of what you're feeling and try to articulate your needs at the end of the exercise.

Complete the following sentences:

1. I am feeling _____.
2. _____ is difficult for me.
3. I need more support when _____.
4. That support might look like _____.

Identify specific action items to help alleviate the emotional blockage, and share what you've written with your partner or your child, depending on the situation. As your child gets older (around three to four years old), this language will also be helpful for him or her to communicate how he or she is feeling and to work toward a solution. My little one has a very difficult time when things are different from what they were expecting or when there are changes to their schedule. Even having their food presented on a different plate or being tucked in with a different blanket can be difficult for them, as are holidays, which are built-up expectations surrounding a day on which the schedule will completely veer from the norm.

Mother's Day Isn't Just Once a Year

Motherhood is one of the most underrated roles in our society. Honestly, I thought it would be a breeze. I spent my twenties traveling the world, starting two businesses, and running an art gallery and an erotic film production company. I was used to working long, hard hours and being pushed to my physical extremes on a daily basis. I thought, *How hard could motherhood really be?*

Don't get me wrong, I love being a mom, but there is no way that I could possibly express to my pre-mommy self the physical, mental, and emotional fortitude that it takes to raise a child and become a parent. One day a year is simply not enough for the celebration of the women who are raising and shaping the next generation of humans. Build time into your week for the mommy time that you need to feel honored, celebrated, and heard. For me, going to yoga or getting a massage or going shopping (without my child) are decadent treats that can help keep me feeling renewed and appreciated. Fill your vessel. When I'm caring for myself, I feel more *me*, and I return home a more relaxed and centered mommy and a more sexually revved up partner.

Time Management

Time management is key to a happy, healthy sex life, and to your overall wellness as a mama and the wellness of your family. First, identify the needs of everyone in the family, and then work out a schedule that caters to the needs and desires of everyone in the family. It might feel like a bummer to schedule intimate time with your partner, but when kids want to play with other kids, do you know what they ask their parents to do? Set up a play date! So set up your own grownup play dates and sculpt erotic adventures with your love.

Weekly Household Meetings

If my partner and I miss our household meeting for the week—which sometimes happens—it is noticeable. The household meeting is a time each week during which you can check in with your partner about your work schedules, the kids' schedules, the sitter's schedule, your emotional needs, date nights, budget and finances, and family goals. You can do any emotional or intimacy check-ins that need to happen and talk about any additional support either of you might need that week. When everyone is on the same page, there are fewer cases of miscommunication throughout the week, and you're less likely to harbor resentment about needs that are left unmet.

Space That Is Yours

It's important for each member of the family to really have a space that is his or her own—whether it's a corner of the family room with a daddy chair and his guitars hung on the wall, or a closet that is converted into a meditation corner with an altar. You can convert a shed in the backyard into a retreat space that is all yours, or maybe just have a special bench under your favorite tree near the tomato plants that you planted. The important thing is creating sacred space that is yours. Retaining space for your own individual self-expression that is separate from your role of mother or partner is essential to the flourishing of a healthy mama's libido and sex life.

A SEXY MAMA'S POV
WITH LUCKY TOMASZEK

When my first baby was born, I knew that I wanted to try to breastfeed her. I wasn't terribly attached to the outcome, though, having heard from a lot of women who experienced lots of difficulties while nursing. Sore nipples, mastitis, low milk supply, baby's food allergies, poor latch—I knew about all of these potential challenges. While I wanted to get through them if they happened to me, I was also open to the option of bottle feeding if breastfeeding became too hard or stressful.

I was really fortunate, though. After an initial weeklong period of pretty intense discomfort right after my babies were born, my breastfeeding experience was physically easy and uncomplicated. I was able to nurse all of my babies into toddlerhood with very few problems.

The one difficulty I had with breastfeeding, and the early years of parenting in general, was sharing my body all the time. (I even experienced this during pregnancy—that inescapable feeling that I had no space of my own.) In addition to nursing my babies, I also wore them in slings and co-slept with them. I believe that babies have a real need for touch and almost constant contact with their caregivers. Our family structured our lives to meet these needs while our kids were little, and allowed them to mature out of it when they were able. It wasn't easy, but the benefits outweighed the drawbacks.

Around three or four months old, breastfeeding babies will start reaching for your face so sweetly. They touch your cheeks and chin, and they want you to kiss their fingers. This is such an endearing time. After so many weeks of putting out physically and emotionally (with little or nothing in return), these expressions of your baby's love feel really good. A couple of months later, as baby gains motor control and strength, these gestures of affection become less gentle and more aggressive.

Babies grow into toddlers, and toddlers grow into preschoolers. This behavior, which starts out so sweet, can grow into a bad habit if left unchecked. We are often so concerned with gentle parenting that we forget to set limits. I have watched mothers tolerate (barely) all sorts of truly unpleasant physical touch from their children: hair twirling, tickling, pinching, patting, nipple flicking, etc. These parents are usually trying to keep the peace while meeting their children's need for touch.

While it's very important to demonstrate empathy and compassion for our children, it's also important to show them how to set limits around their bodies. We do this by setting limits around our own bodies. Our babies are smart, and even when they don't know the meaning of each word we say, they understand our meaning. As long as our message is clear and consistent, babies and toddlers will understand. "I love you very much, but that is my hair (mouth, face, nipple) and I don't want you to touch it right now" is an appropriate statement to make. Not only does this (eventually) end the behavior that is making mom or dad crazy, it also models consent for young children. It establishes a consent culture in your home that will be the foundation for all of your child's relationships outside the family as well.

11

Modeling a Healthy Attitude toward Sex and Self-Care

I KNOW THAT FOR me as a parent, perhaps the most difficult task is to prioritize any type of self-care. Prior to motherhood, I viewed acts of self-care as overly indulgent and a luxury for the privileged that catered to weakness. Working through the difficult stuff without reprieve cultivated my survivor self, my tough, I-can-get-through-anything self.

But it's amazing what motherhood can do to a person. I was told that motherhood would change me. When I heard these words time and time again, I thought folks were referring to my libido or my ability to be an artist or to work within the realm of sexuality. But motherhood changed me in a different way. The moment I discovered I was pregnant, I then had something greater than me to serve, something that was living inside me, and the only way to cater to that thing's needs was to listen to my own body and care for myself.

Throughout the book, we address different ways in which we can identify, articulate, and meet our needs. We have discussed ways in which we can celebrate and honor ourselves by caring for our minds, bodies, and spirits. One of the reasons that this is so necessary is to prevent ourselves from becoming void of energy, passion, and life. Life is simply more fulfilling when we are operating from a place where we are not only sending out love and compassion but receiving it in return. But besides being an essential element of our health and wellness, when we care for ourselves, we are modeling to our children how to advocate for their own well-being and how to embrace self-care.

When our children see us prioritize getting up every morning before the alarm goes off to go for a jog because it makes our bodies feel good and our minds more clear and present, we are teaching our children that they should listen to their bodies and to experiment with how moving their bodies and being active makes them feel. When we institute rituals for self-care, such as starting and ending "quiet time" with a timed two-minute meditation during which mommy's body is not to be touched, we teach our children how to create rituals that aid in our well-being, how to ease transitions with rituals, and how to commit to boundaries around touch and bodies. When we carve out time to make art or write or express ourselves creatively and honor our work as artists in front of our children, it teaches our children to explore modes of creative expression to tell their own stories and express how they are feeling on the inside. When we take wellness days and head off to the beach, we teach our children that taking time out of our schedules to invest in our wellness is just as important as taking time to rest when we are sick.

Remember, not only are we taking care of ourselves, but also, in everything that we do—the way we live our lives and care for our bodies and emotional needs, the way we express our sexual desires, the way we nurture and nourish our relationships and cultivate love for ourselves and others—we are modeling for our children a new attitude toward bodies, toward sexuality, toward intimacy and consent and our own self-worth. We are teaching our children that we are beautiful just as we are, and that they are too. That if we touch any mucous membrane—our nostrils, our mouth, our rectum, or our vulva—we need to wash our hands, and that if we touch our own bodies, it may feel good, and that pleasure is a positive thing in this world. That pleasure is not limited to specific acts, and that the way we share affection, love, and intimacy with one another is also not limited to specific acts but depends on the individual. We are raising sex-positive and body-positive children who will have the language to navigate what is still a very sex-negative society. But these children will be armed with confidence and information, with a positive sense of self and tools to unpack the emotional baggage that they pick up along the way in life. They will find that it is okay to talk about sex, feelings, relationships, intimacy, compassion, desires, needs, and boundaries, because they are already gaining practice in these skillsets starting from the time they are born. Your confidence and well-being, your self-awareness and self-care, are a guide for your children. The environment we create for ourselves and for our children to address bodies and sexuality can either facilitate the acknowledgment of sexuality and intimacy as a natural part of life's journey, or invoke and perpetuate the sexual shame and fear that are reinforced through much of mainstream media and through the puritanical streak that has been embedded deep within our society for generations. It's time to create radical change within ourselves and for our children. It's time for us to step up and be supermodels—or at least super role models—for our children by embracing our whole selves and nurturing our sexual selves like it counts—because it does, and you do.

ON MEETING OUR NEEDS FOR INTIMACY AND CONNECTION
WITH NATASHIA FUKSMAN, MA

When women come in and talk with me, sometimes they'll come in wanting to talk about intimacy with their partner. What they eventually realize, after an initial exploration, is that getting in touch with themselves makes any other intimate relationship much clearer down the line. Start out by looking at your own belly postpartum, honoring it, learning how to see it, and just regularly recognizing the sorts of thoughts that surface. Just commune with the new shape and form of your belly and your vagina. There are many women who come to my new-mom support group who feel they are ready to talk about sex with their partner, but say they haven't looked "down there" yet. So finding what is pleasurable with yourself, by yourself, then taking some very slow steps with partners to rediscovering yourself—it's challenging! For the woman who's been sexually active and then has her first child, for her to have to relearn how to slow down is a process, right? It makes sense to think, "Oh, I just got off the bike, I'll get on again." But it's a process! Our bodies are organic entities in and of themselves, and our minds have shifted so much since having children. Certain things can be eternally more thrilling than they ever were before, but we have to slow down to realize that, as opposed to going on autopilot for the "quickie." Which is not a horrible thing! But it can be an incredibly profound experience to rethink touch with yourself or your partner, like you're learning each other all over again. Give yourself permission to slow down, to masturbate. To gain a real understanding of the process of connecting with your body after this major change takes a while, and that's totally fine and okay. It's not all about waiting by any means.

12

Getting to Know Your New Sexual Self (Exercises)

BEFORE WE CAN GIVE anything to others—whether that's time and attention to our children or intimacy and pleasure to our partners—we must first examine ourselves and get to know our own sexual desires and needs. Without this knowledge we cannot communicate what we need and want and crave, and meeting and fulfilling our undefined needs and desires remains a nearly impossible task.

Intimacy Exercise: Letter Writing

Get out your pen and paper. It's time to write some letters.

Let's start off by writing a letter to your partner about a fantasy that you would like to explore. What is it that you desire that you would like to explore with your partner? How can you ask for what you want? Take five minutes to compose a letter in which you ask your partner for that experience. This might look something like:

> *Dear Lucie,*
>
> *I love you so much. You always inspire me in every way, including in bed. I would really love to explore some new sexual adventures with you. Specifically, I've been thinking that it would be so much fun to experiment with anal pleasure. I would really love to feel your tongue*

on my asshole and have you massage my anus with your lubed-up, gloved fingers. Wow! That would be so hot for me. Maybe we could even find a butt plug to play with. Can we pick it out together? I trust you and love you and can't wait to explore these new aspects of my sexuality with you.

Love,
Tanya

You can delve as deep into the graphic and erotic elements of storytelling as you like in describing your fantasy. Notice what comes easily. What is difficult? How do you feel emotionally as you are writing the letter?

Now, take five minutes and write about the same fantasy, but as if it has already happened. In this letter, you will write to your partner and describe in detail what turns you on about the fantasy as you and your partner might have lived it out last night or last week. An example of this might look like:

Dear Lucie,

Wow! I'm still quivering with pleasure from the insanely hot night that we had. I'm tingling all over! I'm so glad that we decided to get a hotel room and get an overnight sitter. It was so good to just have space for us—I needed that. I needed the whole night with you with no interruptions. I felt so open and vulnerable exposed to you like that, my ass in the air and your mouth up against my puckering anus. God, I'm getting hot just thinking about it! I loved the sound of you snapping on your black latex gloves just before lubing up your hand and filling my ass with your fingers. You made me come so hard! I couldn't keep my hands away from my cunt. I think we're going to need to make this a regular thing. Our monthly mamas' night out. So many more sexual adventures to be had, my love!

Love,
Tanya

After writing about the fantasy in past tense, think about how you felt while writing. How are you feeling in your body right now? Was this second letter easier or more difficult? Many people often find that writing about their fantasy as if it has already happened feels easier and more celebratory. It's an experience that has already happened in your mind, and not an experience that you are asking permission for. Writing about the fantasy in past tense should offer some excitement and arousal while eliminating some of the anxiety. After you have visualized your experience of getting a sitter, going to a hotel, and living out your fantasy, it's much easier to feel empowered to articulate your fantasy and manifest it in real life.

Homework: Choose at least one element of your fantasy letter to manifest. Share your fantasy with your partner. You can always read the letter to your partner and invite him or her to try the letter-writing exercise too! If there are logistics involved, like buying a butt plug or booking a hotel and sitter, make sure to mark your calendar and sort out when you will go sex-toy shopping or research and book a hotel. If your fantasy is too large-scale to live out right now, find a way to take an element of the fantasy and manifest it in real life. Maybe the first step to your anal fantasy, based on the level of energy and sleep the two of you are operating on, is watching some feminist porn with an anal focus after your little one is in bed, and pleasuring one another or pleasuring yourselves together while watching.

Intimacy Exercise: Sensory Play

Set up a "sensory table" with objects to arouse your senses; these can include berries, chocolate, a feather, a leather strap, a strand of hemp rope, a silk scarf, or whatever you like. Close your eyes or have your partner blindfold you. Have your partner wrap his or her body around yours and present the objects for tasting, touching, and exploring with your mouth (your tongue, your lips) or your skin. As your partner presents an object, he or she should gift it with energy and an intention, e.g.: "I'd like to gift you with sweet juicy love and joy of life that I'm sending to your heart (or *your cunt* or *the tips of your toes*)." "Would you like to receive my gift with your mouth?" You can respond, "Yes, please." (A "No, thank you" is always okay too!) Or "I'd like to gift you with a soft caress of sensuality on your nipples. Would you like to receive my gift?", and so on. You can modify the words to something that feels natural to you. Slow things way down. There is no rush. Breathe and really open your heart and your body to receiving touch. This exercise gives you space and time to explore sensation in your pregnant or new-mama body and allows you lots of space to feel that sensation, to feel the energy and connection between you and your partner. As your partner gifts you with love and intention and sensation, really work on taking in that energy, that intention, that love, that is transferred by the object and through your partner's vessel and body to yours. Feel that energy and connection, that tether, and allow it to grow. Exhale any thoughts that go beyond this moment. Come back to your center and release any judgments, insecurities, or chatter in your head. Acknowledge them and let them go. They're keeping you from pleasure and from truly being in this very moment. Feel yourself fill with happiness and compassion. Use your breath to inhale the sensation, the intention, the energy and intimacy flowing from your partner and exhale your gratitude, acceptance, and love of the moment and of your bond. Your body is this brilliant vessel to contain love, to transmit love from one to another. That is intimacy. That is connection.

A RAD DAD'S POV

WITH TOMAS MONIZ *The first time I saw her, she wore a purple bikini. I remember how she strutted by me. I remember how it seemed to barely fit her body, the way her boobs bulged out of the top. I hadn't really been with that many people, and the ones I had been with were more girl than woman; she was a woman.*

The first time we undressed in front of each other a few weeks later, laughing and playful, like only eighteen- and nineteen-year-olds could be, she told me not to call them boobs, that the word made it sound like she was a mother.

"Call them tits," she said.

I said, "I'll call them anything you want. Just please let me hold them."

I often say that with her, I changed from a boy to a man. I learned how to ask rather than expect; I learned to listen rather than talk; I learned about the importance of self-care, boundaries, and consent. I learned how to make love and to fuck.

And, nine months after we hooked up, I learned to be a father.

It's been over twenty years, two more children, a break-up, and a commitment to co-parenting, but I still remember fondly those deliriously giddy and horny prenatal months watching that sexy young thing in the purple bikini transform into the pregnant woman who I lovingly pushed up a hill because she couldn't make it on her own.

And after all this time, I still remember the sex, because it became like a temporary autonomous zone. We threw out everything we knew and had to adapt, rein-vent, rediscover. And sexual exploration is nothing if not hot! We took the time to examine desire and slow down; we learned to talk, to check in. I learned about sex as a multitude of things, rather than a goal or a single act. It was petting and dirty talk and mutual masturbation; it was rubbing oil on the perineum and reminding her how powerful she was; it was discovering which positions worked for her to reach her clit while we fucked around her belly, which seemed to act like a barricade in the bed.

As her body changed, our conversations evolved, just as our sexual positions did. I'd whisper under the covers, "Are they tits or boobs tonight?"—linguistic foreplay to see *whether she felt like a slutty little dirty girl or a soft and sensual mama. Or something else entirely. The options, once you begin talking, are myriad.*

Personally, as the non-birthing partner, I explored the wide spectrum of being sexually intimate with someone, and as a result I discovered how to be a better lover, both to my partner and myself.

As I was telling my best friend about this essay over a beer, I realized that I might never have sex with a pregnant woman again. He commiserated. He has three kids too, and he agreed that there was something both so tender and so wild about sex with your pregnant partner. Something you can't fake.

As I recalled the three periods of pregnant sex with my partner, I realized they were indeed the hottest, dirtiest, most vulnerable and intimate sex moments I'd had. We raised a glass in remembrance. He, of course, in a typical attempt to find a brighter side to things, informed me (as if it would lessen the sting), "There's hella pregnant porn out there, though!"

If I could speak to all the new non-birthing parents, I'd say to use those powerfully intimate nine months when things are changing, foreign, and unfamiliar—perhaps even scary, because she is seeing her own body differently—to talk about sex, desires, and fantasies, openly and honestly. To reinvent yourselves. To pretend that you are starting again, just learning about each other, what she likes, how she likes to be touched.

To ask: Does she like them called titties or boobies?

Role-Playing

WE ARE COMPLEX CREATURES. We are more than just one thing, and when we become parents, we don't give up all of who we are to become a parent. However, the entry into parenthood is a *huge* transition. And transitions can be tricky. They can be complicated and scary. As parents, we haven't lost all the parts of who we are. We haven't ceased to be writers or artists or doctors, or given up our love for sex or rock and roll now that we are parents. But we have gotten a huge new bundle of responsibilities, and our priorities have radically shifted to accommodate for the needs of a tiny new human who relies on us for everything. When the way we spend our days changes so drastically—from caring from our own needs to caring for the needs of someone else—it can challenge our perception of self and our identity.

Who are we, now that we are parents? What parts of my self-care and sexual identity carry over from my pre-mommy life, and what parts of my identity are newly forming? There is a period during which we are getting to know ourselves again. It's a curious time. How do we meet our own needs when we are grappling to figure out what that might look like now that we are parents?

I know for me, I felt panicky during this period of not knowing. I didn't like the unknown variables and not having a clear vision of the future me that I was becoming. But I kept reminding myself to be gentle and slow with myself. I was generally managing dozens of projects at a time pre-motherhood, but I was lucky to accomplish even one thing on my action list each day while I was nursing my little one. Change is a constant, but drastic change can be difficult. Especially if it is not what we are expecting.

So how do we get to know our partners as parents and as lovers now that we are parents? If you are co-parenting with your partner, you might find that your relationship has shifted from a romantic one to one that is more utilitarian as you both work to meet all your baby's needs. Tensions can arise if one partner feels that the other is not as involved or not working as hard at nurturing and caring for the child. There might be jealousy surrounding the self-care that one parent is getting, but not the other. There are many different relationship dynamics and tensions that can arise during this time of transition, as parents are settling into their child-nurturing roles and discovering their own newly evolved identities as individuals and as a couple.

If you start to experience a strong emotion like jealousy—whether it's jealousy of the attention that the new baby is receiving or of the self-care that your partner is engaging in—I've learned that it helps to name it, identify it, and explore it a little more. Give your emotion room to talk. Journaling, self-talk, or therapy are all great for this. Sometimes I'll give myself space to write and have a dialogue with the emotion. This is not a dialogue with my partner. Wait until to you get to the essence of the problem and solution before clouding your partner's psyche with a release of big distracting emotions. Give yourself space for the emotional offloading and then get to the issue underneath it.

For example:

I'm feeling really pissed.
Why are you feeling pissed?
I'm just so jealous.
Really?
Yeah, did you hear him? He just went biking—by himself—and had lunch—*on his own!*

That sounds really healthy. Like he's taking care of himself.

Yeah! When do *I* get to do that? I was here at the house all day running after our child and was only able to gobble down half a sandwich before running our daughter to the potty and wiping her butt and cleaning the house. When do *I* get to have a break?

Do you need a break?

Yes.

Okay. So it sounds like you really need some space to yourself to decompress and eat on your own and maybe take a walk or a bike ride. Is that right?

Yes.

How about this evening? He's home now and he has eaten and his vessel is full of self-care. Go let him know what you need.

Thanks.

From there I go ask for what I need and take the time I need to decompress. When those emotions come up, it usually means a need isn't being met. I try to work in daily, weekly, and monthly self-care, but life happens, and sometimes schedules can be unpredictable. Forgive yourself and start again. Adapt. Make the changes that you need to fit the self-care you need into your life.Give yourself time and space to release emotion and find what your needs are. Judgments and name-calling and pointed emotions are not needs. They may come up in our minds, but we can acknowledge them, investigate them, and release them.

Forming and Honoring Different Parts of Our Psyche

I was meeting with a new parent couple that I was coaching, and the husband said, "I'm having a hard time thinking of my wife as anything but a mother now. How do we get to a point where we can think of one another as lovers again?"

There are many parts to our psyche, and we are capable of tapping into many of them and developing many different roles to play in this life. Here are some of the roles you may or may not find within yourself but which can all exist simultaneously.

Lover—The passionate, sexy, sensual woman is in there. She is. She might not be the most dominant character in your life during new motherhood, and she might be hungry for attention when your hormones are raging during pregnancy. She doesn't always have to be at the forefront of your psyche, but it's also important to remember that she is there and to spend some time with her. Don't leave her neglected just because your identity is shifting. Find new ways for her to come out and play.

Household manager and activities director—This is the part of your identity that handles coordinating your kids' play dates, mom's groups, grocery shopping, laundry, clean sheets, dishes, menu planning, organizing sitters, and activities for the family. It's where my Virgo self shines! This is a dominant part of my personality—the part of me that likes to have control. It's where the routines and schedules are made.

Mother—This is a complex and ever-evolving part of my identity. What is your mothering self like? Silly? Nurturing? Cuddly? Loving? Enduring? Tender? How does your mothering self dress? Is it different from your Lover self? Are you an earth mama? A wacky artist mama? A rocker mama? A soccer mama? Know that this part of your identity is as unique as you are and will change and evolve as your relationship with your child changes and evolves.

Child—Yes, you do have a child self too! Just because you are now a mom doesn't mean that your identity doesn't include a child that needs to be nurtured; that wants to throw a tantrum when things don't go your way; that needs a big hug, a big cuddle, and to be taken care of occasionally. This is a tender, vulnerable part of ourselves. When we nurture ourselves, we are caring for our child selves as well. My child self loves to color. Your child isn't the only one who can have a box of crayons. More and more studies are coming out revealing the stress-relieving benefits of coloring. So nurture your child self.

Animal—Lions and tigers and bears, oh my! Have you ever growled in bed? Meowed? Do you purr when you're happy? Do you find that when you get excited, you wag your tail like a puppy? We all have these deeply ingrained animal selves, primal parts of our identity. What does your animal self look like? Where does it live in your body? What characteristics does its personality encompass? One of my animal identities is a spaniel puppy—excitable, playful, loyal, affectionate, and a bit messy.

Career woman—If you are balancing a career and motherhood, you might have a part of your identity that is specific to your job and the role that you play there. Are you a manager? Are you service oriented? Do you dress a certain way at work? Speak a certain way? What skills do you utilize in your job? What parts of your personality come out and shine through in your work? What are your work relationships like? Many mothers take at least six weeks off from work postpartum (if not longer). This might be a part of us that morphs dramatically; when we go back to work, we may feel the mothering part of our identity pulling us toward the home. I went back to work only a few weeks after giving birth. I believe it was two weeks after the birth of my little one that I started working on an art exhibition, working part time with my editors on films that were on deadline, and writing essays for anthologies. But honestly, it was too soon for me. I felt a radical loss of self even in being removed from work for two weeks. I was used to truly being defined by my work. Who was I if my work self was gone? I very slowly learned how to create balance in my life. I learned to appreciate stillness and the importance of having space from my work self in order to fuel my creative self and bring focus and presence back to my mothering self. Each individual has to discover where her energies lie and what fuels her in her life at that moment. Motherhood has taught me how to prioritize and consider the energy and time I'll be giving to any individual project, and weigh whether or not that is something that truly makes me happy. Being a mother has made me a smarter career woman.

There are dozens of other facets of our identity that might revolve around the activities that fuel us and make us who we are. We are not just the mother, but the mother is never completely gone from our identity. Just as our other selves are always there.

Role-Playing Game

When my coaching client, who I mentioned above, made that statement about having a hard time viewing his wife as a lover when she seemed engulfed in her identity as a mother, I recommended that the two of them try some role-play.

Role-playing is simply constructing a character or a personality different from the ones you inhabit in your everyday life. You might also choose to create scenarios to play out with these characters. This can be a fun, playful way to step into another part of yourself or create another part to play. It can give you freedom from your own everyday responsibilities and the roles that you find yourself playing. This should be a role that you are excited about stepping into. A role that is tantalizing or empowering or compelling to you; not a role that is placed upon you. You might have absolutely no inclination to be a French maid or a milkman, but maybe you do. Think about what roles and archetypes turn you on. What characters turn you on?

When I was speaking with the couple that I was coaching, it came up that the woman had always felt that librarians were really sexy. I was very excited to hear this, as I have always found the librarian to be an incredibly sexy role as well. I encouraged her to buy a few new wardrobe items. No need to go wild and spend a lot, but there should be a wardrobe for your role. Something that differentiates your everyday self from your role-playing character. She bought some very sexy lacy lingerie; garters and thigh-high stockings; a tight, hip-hugging pencil skirt; and some sheer button-up blouses along with a pair of glasses. She was able to transform herself into the Sexy Librarian, and her husband was able to ask the Sexy Librarian out on a date. It was like he was dating another woman! Her sexual self, and the sexual permission she needed to take charge in her new sexual self, existed in this character. She needed a transitional vehicle to move from the role of mother to lover. What is *your* transitional vehicle to move from mother to lover?

We've talked a bit about the development of parts of yourself that could serve as your "sexual self" that exists outside of your role as parent. This allows you to develop relationships with new parts of yourself. Think about a potential role that might be sexy to explore. Explore the concept of this character as an extension, a part of you that you are exploring in a safe environment. Start to discuss potential fantasies with your partner. Who is this character? What are her desires? How do you think she likes to have sex? What turns this character on? Go shopping for a wardrobe for that character. Does she wear racy lingerie under her pencil skirt? Thigh-high stockings and garters under her conservative outerwear? Play around with your dynamics in this role. You could even go on a date as this character. How does she act? What would she say? Allow this character to be a tool to explore a different part of your psyche—your sexual self—your self outside of your parent self.

Intimacy Exercise: Self-Reflection

Get out a mirror and look at your body. Create space to really look at yourself and love the vessel that you are in, in this moment. Many women have feelings of anxiety around looking at their vulvas during pregnancy or postpartum. Love your vulva as it is. In all its changes. Really take a close look at your body: your vulva. Your belly. What has changed? What has shifted? What is the same? I like to look at my vulva and then lovingly cup my hand over it and give it a little massage, a little rub, a little hug. If you are three months or more postpartum, I also highly recommend getting a plastic speculum (you can buy them online at goodvibes.com). They're only about five dollars! Put glycerin-free lubricant on and around your vulva and inside your vagina, and a little on the speculum. Insert the speculum so that the handle is pointed downward toward your anus, and click the speculum open. With a small flashlight and mirror, you should be able to locate your cervix! That tiny pin of a hole is your cervix, and it's what your little one passes through during birth. Isn't that wild? That is a part of you, and you are beautiful! Now, release the lock and slowly pull out the speculum. If you insert the speculum again with the handle pointed to your left or right and click it open, you will notice a spongy ridged or ruffled tissue on the ceiling of the vagina umbrellaing downward. That is your paraurethral sponge, a glandular tissue also known as the G-spot. If you keep the speculum in and stimulate your clitoris, you will notice that this glandular tissue begins to grow bigger. That's because it is an erogenous zone; it is engorging with blood, as well as swelling with glandular fluid known as ejaculate. Slowly release the lock and remove the speculum. Thank your vulva and give it some love. You just got to know your body on a whole new level.

Homework: With your partner, discuss some characters or archetypes that the two of you might want to role-play. What do the characters wear? What do they look like? What are their personalities like? Create a scenario that you and your partner can play out as these characters. Will you be meeting in public? At a bar? A restaurant? Get playful and discover new roles for your sexual selves to experiment with, and watch the new sexual energy pour in.

A SEXY MAMA'S POV
WITH SHAR REDNOUR

I am the matriarch[1] of a two-mom, multiracial family created through public adoption.[2]

My wife and I were together for eleven years before we became parents, so we had lots of sex before we were moms. I highly recommend doing that. Later, when we were too exhausted to have sex, we didn't turn against each other from insecurity or resentment because we had proof that we were hot for each other. I didn't have to guess or have great self-esteem; I knew that she wanted to do the nasty because that's all we used to do! I've given this advice out in person as well as in books and articles: If you are even thinking of becoming a parent, then screw like

---

1   Although there are two moms, my wife is trans-butch masculine identified, so she wouldn't call herself a matriarch.

2   Public adoption is free. It matches adopting parents to local children whose parents are unable to parent or have died. Oftentimes it's done with a foster-to-adopt program.

crazy. No, not to get pregnant, but to be utterly connected in that altered state of pleasure and orgasm. You will need this intimacy-gasoline in your love tank later when you are parents. Oh yes, your family love tank will be over-flowing, but your couple (or poly) love tank will be zapped, I promise. I'm thrilled when parents seek me out years later to thank me because they listened and had a great time shoring up their relationship before they became parents. I mean, what "homework" could be more fun?

One of the great things about adoption is that you don't start parenting physically exhausted from giving birth (but you do get tired later). You also don't have your lady parts worked over. Hey, you might not even have to do Kegels until you're sixty! Sorry, I joke, but adoption is so rare that I point out any advantages I can in hopes that it helps a child.[3] On the other hand, with regard to sex, one issue is that many adoptive parents believe in holding our babies or new children all the time for bonding. Baby books will tell you to let a relative take care of the baby so you can get some relationship time, but many adoption books do not say this. One of our children cried anytime anyone besides me or Jackie held him. We didn't want him to have one more moment of stress after all he had gone through. We rarely put our baby down, so that made finding sexy "alone time" a little more difficult than it is for folks who send the baby off to grandma's house. We worked in sexy time when he napped. I also nursed our youngest children using Lact-Aid, a system for adoptive mothers to breast-

---

3   As a sex educator, I must clarify my joke for anyone taking me seriously—many women benefit from doing Kegel exercises at any age, whether they've given birth or not.

feed. Unlike birth mothers, I couldn't fall asleep after a feeding; I had to tear myself away to wash out tubes (not immediately, but they clog if you don't do it within a few hours). That was tiring. I gave our kids the benefit of breastfeeding, yet I didn't get some of the benefits, like not having to deal with cleaning.

As the kids grew, we valued time alone (whether in a hotel or our house) as golden. We could get friends to watch the kids while we went out, but we really wanted to stay in without the kids. So we created a co-op movie night with four families. One night a month we had all the kids; then for three Fridays we were free.

As a mother of three boys, I strike a balance between being nurturing and not being a female doormat. It's very difficult. I have to stay in full feminist consciousness and not be on autopilot so I don't fall into the traps of our culture. I want my children to be babied and adored and have a childhood, yet I don't want them confusing women with maids. I hope I'm succeeding, but I can't promise. My answer to almost all issues is honesty. I often say, "We're a family and we work together." But this affects my sex life and relationship when the kids want us to be theirs for the asking twenty-four seven. I stress the importance of mama and I having good couple time. I tell them that Jackie and I are the foundation of the entire family, and that as long as we are strong, the whole family is strong. Now they know it's a value of our family, and they support that value the same way they uphold other family values like sharing food or not calling each other names. They get it. I always joked that having more than one kid is the real polyamory—how can you split your love in that many directions and keep everyone happy? I'm grumpy, lackluster, and stupid when

I haven't connected with Jackie or myself sexually—or, as I like to say, "gotten my hormones balanced." Getting attention from her (or from my vibrator) delivers a hopeful matriarch full of ideas and enough energy to enjoy the special family we've created.

CHAPTER 4

Sexual Exploration Agreements, Games

PERHAPS ONE OF THE greatest hurdles that all couples face, regardless of whether you have a child, is communication. It sounds so easy, doesn't it? Talking isn't so hard. But with all that we study in school, we are given very few actual tools and practice for expressing our emotions and needs in a way that is honest and that nurtures our relationships. And we are given even fewer tools for how to navigate talking about, communicating about, and articulating our sexual needs and desires. It is no wonder that so many women go years without pleasure from their partners, afraid to talk about the sex they want or to seek out the sex and pleasure they desire.

One of the most helpful tools that I've discovered is a very simple one. It's what I call the sexual exploration agreement. In Chapter 7, I had you make an agreement with yourself. Now I'd like for you to make an agreement with your partner. This is a changing, living, breathing document. It will not stay static, as we do not stay static. It will act as a simple or complex container for you and your partner to state your desires, needs, and what you would like to commit to exploring, and to access how nurturing those things made you feel. What worked for you and what didn't.

I recommend making the agreement for a very short time period when you first start out, and then you can extend it with a check-in once a month. Always set a review date when creating the agreement, and try not to be overambitious. Start slowly and add to it. This is not a race. There are no winners or losers. This is all about just nurturing you and your partner in your relationship and communicating with one another about your sexual desires. The conversations surrounding the agreement and the reflection and revision time are just as important as the agreement itself.

This can really look like whatever works for you, but here is a basic form to start with. The purpose is to have a single container for holding things you may want to explore in your relationship, boundaries you may have, desires you want to manifest, things that will serve your relationship, and commitments you are making to the wellness of your unity.

Make a Sexual Exploration Agreement

1. State your needs and desires in this relationship.
2. State your partner's needs and desires.
3. List the fantasies you would like to commit to exploring, and state how long you will commit to this (a week? a month?).
4. Explore how these fantasies will manifest in your everyday life. For example: *Once a month we will go to a sexuality workshop that interests us. At least twice a week, I will place a note of love and gratitude in my partner's mailbox.*

   Or, *On Date Night Friday, I won't wear any panties, and I'll wear the high heels that you always drool over.*

   Or, *Every Friday night we will have a date night, even if that means pitching a tent in our backyard and making out over toasted marshmallows after the kids are asleep.*

Treat this document as a working agreement that you both nurture and refer back to on a monthly basis. If something isn't working, find out why and change it. The agreement should be used as a communication tool. If it feels obligatory, it needs to change. Leave room for change and acknowledge that change is okay. What you desire will change. There are no rules for what your relationship has to look like. Set an expiration date for review and revision.

COMMUNICATING WITH OUR PARTNERS
WITH NATASHIA FUKSMAN, MA

In our culture, for people who are spiritually inclined, whether through a particular religion or not, premarital counseling is seen as a regular part of getting married. I think it would be a wonderful thing if we began a cultural shift toward couples counseling before you have a baby. Going to see a couples counselor who's really versed in the transitions of parenthood and in talking about sex can really help a couple develop some ground rules and safety measures, as well as help them talk about sex when a female partner is pregnant. Someone who is really well trained can help ease the weight a little bit on how to have those conversations with one another, how to accept each other, and even how to learn the words to suss out touch, sex, visual appeal, and desire. It can be infinitely helpful way beyond the first year postpartum.

Let's Play a Game!

Grownups can play games too! Games are just another way that individuals connect with one another. So let's play a few of our own games. Before trying any of the games in this chapter, make sure to set your terms and outline your boundaries, limits, and rules. Reserve the right to call a timeout to step out of the game and revise the rules if it's going in a direction that isn't sexy or that you are not enjoying. Remember, games are meant to be fun and should be something that both parties consent to, not something they feel obligated to engage in. Have fun! Break the ice and explore your new, sexy desires in a playful way.

Sexy Game Ideas and Prompts:

These are just a few of my favorites to play. Feel free to create your own games too!

I Spy—Look around the room and find something that turns you on or reminds you of a sexual fantasy, desire, or memory. Then say to your partner "I spy with my little eye something that turns me on, and the color is..." (Or "it smells like..." or "it tastes like...") Try to get your senses engaged. Then your partner can start guessing and you can start giving hints. Take turns playing this back and forth. This can be a fun game to play when you're out on date night and waiting for dinner to arrive, or really any time! Get playful and spy something that turns you on.

Once Upon a Time—Choose a fairy tale and kink up the story to an adult level. Goldilocks and the Three Perverts is one of my favorites.

Remote Control Fantasies—Get a remote-controlled vibrator and hand the remote over to your partner during your date. It can be wildly exciting to be out in public and secretly be stimulated by your partner, trying to contain your pleasure. Good Vibrations (goodvibes.com) is an excellent source for remote-controlled vibes.

Twister—Get an old Twister game and play with your partner. This is a great way to be silly and physical with each other as your bodies intertwine. Want to sex it up? Try Twister in your undies, or naked! You can also add body parts to the spinner. Right hand to left breast. Tongue to cock. Lips to cunt. The possibilities are endless.

Wrestling—Playful wrestling, much like Twister, can be both physical and erotic. It's a physical activity that gets our adrenaline pumping and our energy up and gets us back into our bodies. This is also an activity that you can sex up by removing layers of clothing. Makes sure that there is plenty of negotiation prior to wrestling. Also, wrestling is likely not something you'll want to do during your pregnancy or directly after giving birth—at least not full-body wrestling. Full-body wrestling is something that will require some padding on the floor and conscious-ness around bodies. This is more an exploration of energy and force and power melding back and forth. Negotiations beforehand are a must. Play safe. And yes, we can bring some of this dynamic into pregnancy and the postpartum period. Do you remember the days of thumb wrestling and arm wrestling? This can be such a fun chance to physically connect with your partner in a playful way. You can also play for different fun and sexy things: "Best two out of three wins. If I win, I get a massage and a spanking. If you win you get a long, slow blow job." Each person should decide what he or she is playing for; all acts should be sexy things that the two of you would love to engage in whether you win or lose, so that everyone is a winner.

Kinky Simon Says—Simon says take off your shirt. Simon says unzip your pants. Simon says pull out your strap-on cock. Stick your cock in my mouth. I didn't say "Simon Says!"

Secret Sexy Word of the Day—Do you remember on *Pee-wee's Playhouse* how at the beginning of each episode Pee-wee would tell us the secret word of the day, and then whenever someone said that word during the episode Pee-wee and everyone in the house would scream playfully? The sexy version of this is: When someone says _____ (choose a word), you _____ (something sexy or romantic). This is a fun game to play in public. Decide on a word, and if you hear the word while you are out on your date, then you will do something sexy. Maybe you'll take off your panties in public. Maybe you'll make out with your partner or put your hand down your partner's pants or up your own skirt! It's important that this is negotiated in such a way that it's mutual and that both partners are excited, turned on, and titillated by the activities.

Truth or Dare—This game doesn't really even need to be modified from its original version. Revisit your teen years and connect intimately and physically with your partner over a game of Truth or Dare. Even after being together for years, you can always discover new things about your partner or dare one another to complete sexy challenges. Again, as with any of these games, discuss limits and boundaries beforehand and always reserve the right to mid-game negotiations, but also keep an open mind and remember that this is a tool for articulating your desires and connecting intimately with your partner.

Time for a Field Trip!—Get out of the house! Find a sitter. Trade nights with another parent. Go explore the world outside the house with your partner. It's time for a field trip. Just because you are now a parent (or pregnant) doesn't mean that the sexual adventures have come to an end. This is a brand-new chapter of your lives to experience. How exciting is that? So even if your pre-mommy life didn't involve going to erotic film festivals or shopping for sex toys with your partner, it doesn't mean that can't be a part of your new sexy mama life. Discover what you are now passionate about. What turns you on? Sample the erotic delicacies of the world through a whole new lens. Do bookstores turn you on? Go make out among the bookshelves. If art is what gets you going, make out at a museum among beautiful paintings. Do you love nature? Go visit the redwood trees and explore nature in a whole new way, taking in the scents and textures of the wild while connecting intimately with your partner.

I know for me, I also feel a whole new gratitude and appreciation for the time that my partner and I get to spend together. We appreciate our alone time even more now that we are parents, and our intimacy and desire for one another has grown more and more over the years.

Erotic film festivals are becoming more and more popular. Being out in public with your partner and watching super hot sex on screen can get the juices flowing. Can't wait for an erotic film festival to come your way? Go out to a sexy movie. A grownup movie. One without animation. A night out at the movie theater can be so much fun. See a foreign film or an arthouse film, something that turns you both on. Feel that sexy energy between the two of you and try to engage in touch in the theater—hands touching in the popcorn box; hands on thighs or making their way into pants. Going to the movies brings out my horny teenage self that wants to do dirty things in the dark theater. Maybe it will bring out some unexpected erotic characteristics in you too!

Go to a sex-positive toy store and pick out some new toys for your sexual adventures. Don't have a sex-toy store in your city? See what kinky and sexy pervertables you and your partner can find at your local hardware store, kitchen supply store, dollar store, or pet store! For about six months, when my child was one year old, our family relocated out to the desert in San Bernardino. It was a brief experience but a difficult one. And there definitely weren't any sex-positive sex-toy stores where we were living—but there was a Home Depot! We found so many erotic implements there to satiate our kinky lives. Or just look around your house for pervertables. This morning I had a wonderful post-breakfast spanking from my partner with a spatula while our little one was sleeping. Enjoy the small connected moments.

Slip into Something Sexy—Go shopping with your partner for lingerie! Or heels, or anything else that makes you feel sexy. This has a huge impact on my libido. While I was pregnant, my body was changing dramatically, but I refused to forfeit my lingerie for blah, functional underthings. As my body changed, I bought new lingerie, lace bras and panties, slips, garters, stockings, and more! You don't have to spend a lot. I especially love to go to vintage stores for slips. The important thing is finding clothes that make you feel confident and sexy. I found that finding the right wardrobe was also very important for me in my postpartum transformation into my sexy mama self. I loved garters and waist cinchers and even vintage girdles and corsets. It made me feel more confident about my belly that was still shrinking and tiger-striped. I learned to love my tiger stripes, but it was nice to have options. I also found some sexy nursing bras at Hot Milk. I find that shopping can be especially sexy with my partner, because then I get to model my favorite lingerie pieces—and depending on the privacy of the dressing room, you and your partner might fit in a little foreplay and sexy time too!

Be Naked Together—Try sleeping naked with your partner. It's amazing how just losing that thin layer of clothing between the two of you and having your naked bodies close to one another under the sheets can make everything feel so much more sensitive and can even be a catalyst for middle-of-the-night sex or morning sex with your sweetie.

Visit the Hot Tubs—Many hot tub facilities have private rooms, which means you and your partner can have privacy—something that can feel like a rare and coveted treat when you become a parent. You can engage in sexy time and get a chance to soak and relax.

Go Dancing—Get out on the dance floor. Try a new type of dance— ecstatic dance, burlesque, ballroom dancing, African dance, or even twerking (not my style, but some of my sexy mama friends are totally into it!). Just get out there and move your bodies—and when you can, move your bodies together. I wouldn't say that I'm a great dancer. In fact, I pretty much have two left feet, I'm pretty clumsy and uncoordinated. You don't have to be a talented dancer to move your body to music. Find a type of dance or movement that gets you back into your body and feeling physical.

Make Art Together—I met my partner when he was a photographer and I was a model, and I feel deeply connected to him on both a romantic and an artistic level. When I have the opportunity to make art with him, it's ecstatic. When we became parents, we lost some of that artist/collabo- rator relationship, so now we make art dates together. It's a way that we further that intimate connection that we have together. Write a story with your partner, paint together, build something together, or learn to cook together. Art can be a really sexy mode of self-expression, and so intimate. Try collaborating with your partner on a project. You might just find that your artistic passion leads to a whole new level of love and inti- macy that has you pawing at one another like horny art-school students.

Homework: Write notes for your partner in places where he or she will find them. A book he or she is reading, on his or her laptop, on the package of cookies that he or she always reaches for after work. Sticky notes are great for this so that the note doesn't float away. I also like to do this with sexy Polaroid self-portraits with a little note on them. Finding little reminders and notes all around the house that express how much you are loved and desired and how much you turn your partner on can fill your vessel and deepen connection and be a catalyst for hot steamy sex between you and your love.

A SEXY MAMA'S POV
WITH LUCKY TOMASZEK

I had my first baby when I was twenty-two years old. Despite my relatively young age, I had always known that I wanted to be a mom as soon as possible. Those early months of parenthood were unspeakably difficult, as they almost always are. I was exhausted and depressed. My husband and I decided that it would be best for everyone if I stayed home full time. Though it's not for everybody, I really loved being home with my baby. I felt settled and fulfilled, something I wouldn't have imagined for myself in all those years of adolescent turbulence immediately preceding motherhood. But it was also isolating and frustrating, only ever talking to someone who couldn't talk back.

Sexually speaking, this period following my baby's birth was full of other kinds of discoveries. It took a long while for my drive to return. Never in my life had I been so disinterested in sex. I didn't feel negative about it; I just didn't feel anything about it at all. But when the mood did strike me, I realized that my orgasms were far more intense than they had been before. They swept over more of my body, and took me further into space than ever before. I also felt a deeper attachment to my husband during sex than I ever had. Our time together in the birth room, and raising this new little person as partners, strengthened our bond. Before, our sex had been really good, and often very fun. Now our sex brought us together in a new way. This meant that, although sex was less frequent, it was better than ever.

This diminished drive coupled with increased sexual response happened after each of our babies. Each birth taught me more about the power of my body and put me in touch with my sex organs in a deeper and more profound way. I learned to read myself closely, and figured out how to intensify my orgasms even more by contracting certain groups of my PC muscles at certain times.

All told, I spent about ten years either pregnant, breastfeeding, or both. In those years, I spent countless nights holding and rocking fussy infants and toddlers. I shared my body and my bed with feverish, teething, cranky, mischievous, intelligent little ones for that entire decade. Like all parents, I learned how to continue swaying and shushing well past the point of exhaustion, and how to sleep in truly uncomfortable positions to keep the baby asleep. I learned how to hold the space for someone else's emotional outbursts and help them feel secure in my love, no matter what else was happening.

These skills are part and parcel of parenting, of course. But I was astonished by the way they translated to being a better lover. When I am pleasing my partner, I can tune into them and focus in a way that would have been impossible before kids. I gained so much physical strength, stamina, and empathy as a direct result of those beautiful, difficult years. Those are gifts that I continue to be grateful for, even all these years later.

15

Let's Go on a Date!

I CAN'T EMPHASIZE ENOUGH the importance of date nights. Date nights need not be for only you and your partner, but can also include your child. Or it can be a date for yourself, or—if you and your partner are polyamorous—dates with other people.

But now that you have a kid, there is a little more work involved in crafting a date night. It's not as simple as "Hey, let's catch a movie tonight"—there is the whole issue of finding a sitter or care for your child.

In this chapter you will find some tips guiding you through how to craft a date night, along with challenges you might encounter and ways to overcome them, save the cherished date night, and nurture time for yourself and your relationships with others.

Date Night (No Sitter—Kiddo Makes Three or More!)

So you have probably been there. It's the weekend and you were hoping to go out for a night on the town with your sweetie, but every babysitter in town is already booked! Fear not, mamas—you can still go out for a date night with your kid(s).

Of course, it will be different from a night on the town with just the two of you, but you can still make time to connect with your love. Opt for an early-ish dinner date after you have already fed your munchkin.

Depending how old your little one is, maybe you'll have him or her asleep in the stroller while you and your partner share a pizza and a beer, or catch an outdoor movie screening at the park, or eat from food trucks while listening to local bands play at an all-ages venue or space that is accommodating for children.

I generally find that restaurants or music venues with outdoor seating make for an easy getaway if your little one wakes up or you need to head home for some reason. I live in California, so there are a lot of outdoor spaces here, but if you live in an area of the country that gets cold during the winter, you can find a favorite diner to bring baby along to where you can share a milkshake and a piece of pie and put quarters in the jukebox or play arcade games over vegan hot dogs and beer. You could go bowling or putt-putt golfing or head to a late-night art museum event.

Also, outdoor venues tend to be all-ages. You might have a baby in a sling, nursing or sleeping against you, but that doesn't mean you can't still enjoy a movie, hold hands, make out, and have a romantic date out in the world with your love, enjoying each other and getting the quality date night time that you need.

When dating with kids, we just know that we must expect the unexpected. Cherish each moment and know that stuff happens. There will be times when your child simply won't go to sleep or is teething or sick. Just as you have off days, so will your little one, and you must accommodate for that and take care of one another. The date might be cut short, and that is okay. Parenting has taught me truly to savor the moment.

Date Night (Grown-Ups only)

Woohoo! So you got grandma to watch your wee one or a sitter or a friend to be your childcare resource for the evening. Congrats! Now what? When I'm planning a date night with my love, I try to think about a few things: When? How much energy and money should we expend? What is going on? What do we both need?

When?—Some people like to put date nights on the calendar on the same day each week, or every other week. For me it works better to be flexible, based on whether I'm interested in a low-key weeknight date or an exciting, energy-packed weekend nighttime adventure date. If we are going out on a weekend, there is going to be a lot of commotion and energy surrounding us. We live in the Bay Area, and on the weekend everyone is going out to dinner or a show. There are a lot of festivals and events and a lot of drinking going on. It takes a fair amount of energy even to engage with or make our way through a restaurant on the weekend. It's generally going to be a louder date. These aren't necessarily negatives, but it's something to be aware of when planning. Will you have the energy to go out to see a band at a rock venue or go to a fetish club on Saturday night? Or will you be depleted from lack of sleep and a stressful work week and need to opt for something more low-key like your favorite pizza parlor and soaking in a hot tub on a Wednesday evening?

How much energy and money should we expend?—Dates can be as expensive or cheap as you want them to be. Date night doesn't have to mean going out to a fancy restaurant every week with your love. It's about the time that you're sharing together. So whether it's going to a free concert in the park or having hot cocoa and reading poetry to one another at your favorite coffee house, your date should be something that nourishes you and your partner, creating time and space dedicated for connection and intimacy. Check in with yourself and your partner about budget and how much energy you both have based on what else is going on in your lives that week. I like to book our date nights at our weekly household meetings, while we are also reviewing our finances and schedules for the upcoming week. It makes for an easy time to figure out what kind of date might best fit our lives that week.

What is going on?—Checking out calendars for your favorite venues, theaters, or communities can be a great way to book your date nights. What is going on that is exciting and interesting and sexy to you in the city or town that you live in? Is there a cooking class, a couples dance class, a fellatio or bondage workshop? Find the pulse of what is going on where you live and let it be a springboard for putting dates on your calendar.

What do we both need?—One of you might have a lot of energy and be dying to get out in the world, while the other just wants to have a relaxing evening. Make sure both of your needs are being met. Sometimes we need to go on dates by ourselves, or with friends or other partners. Make time to meet your own needs. Ultimately you will feel more fulfilled, have your needs met, and come home a healthier, more renewed version of you. Fill your vessel, and you will bring that energy to your relationship with your child and your partner.

Date Night (Night In)

If you don't have the resources to go out for a date, you can always stay in! Wait until after bedtime and have a movie date with your partner. Rent a movie from iTunes, pop some popcorn, and snuggle up close to your sweetie. You can also have a late-night dinner or dessert together over a glass of wine, or have a bondage date post-bedtime. Just because you are staying in doesn't mean your sex life has to be boring. Get creative and woo your partner inside your house.

Date Night Makeover and Assessment

Answer these questions and start to sculpt your dream sexy mama dating life.

- What words would you choose to describe a dream date night with your partner?
- What are the places where you feel the most connected to your partner?
- Describe a recent date night experience where you had an incredible time.

Before going out on your date, consider the following:

- How full is your vessel? What is your energy level?
- Where will your date happen?
- What will your date consist of?
- What are your expectations?

- What energy level is needed? How do you plan to prepare yourself, energetically and emotionally?
- What are elements that cue your feeling of love and connection on a date?
- What annoys you during a date? What are your limits?

And after the date, ask yourself:

- What is your rose? And your thorn? (These are expressions my child and I use, and I use them in all my relationships now. Your "rose" is something really lovely that happened during your date, and your "thorn" is something that was challenging or difficult.)

Homework: Plan a date for this week. Consider what you and your partner need most right now, your energy levels, and how and where you might best connect. Write it down and put it on your calendar. If what you need most right now is a date with yourself or with your friends, schedule that instead.

16

Spicing Up Your Sex Life as a Parent

WHEN I THINK ABOUT spicing up the bedroom and truly carving out time for intimate moments and hot sex, I think about creativity. Parenthood teaches us to be in the moment, to plan ahead, and to think outside of the box. The creative sexual scenarios that parenthood has inspired for me remind me of my early sexual experiences when I was eighteen and nineteen with my first girlfriends and boyfriends. We got so creative regarding where and how to have sex. A bed was not a necessity, and in fact was mostly a luxury, especially when I was living with my mom. There was car sex, cheap hotel sex, public bathroom sex, movie theater blow jobs, and making out on picnic blankets. We never seemed to run out of places to find intimate connection.

As a parent, I don't hide my affection for my partner. We kiss, hug, snuggle, and are physically close to one another in front of our little one. I think it is important to model a loving, consenting, affectionate relationship. We let our child know when she knocks or walks in when we are making love that we need space and privacy, and we let our child know that she can always ask for space and privacy when she needs it too. And she does ask for it, and we make sure to give her the space she needs. Each parent, of course, must access their own comfort with talking about sex, intimacy, consent, and privacy with their children. We will address that in Chapter 18.

But thinking outside of the box and outside of the bedroom can be really advantageous for us as parents. Think about where you get the space and privacy that you need or desire to explore your body, pleasure, and connection with your partner. In the shower? If so, maybe you need to put together a sex kit for the bathroom and keep it on mommy's shelf. A waterproof vibrator, a detachable showerhead—what do *you* need in the bathroom to increase your pleasure? For me, a big part of sexing up the shower was having shower gel in a scent that I really enjoy and luxurious lotion to rub all over my body, as well as a silk robe that feels sexy and sensuous against my body. Maybe the living room couch is where you and your partner like to get intimate. Figure out what you might need and have it in a nearby, accessible spot. I keep my lube, nipple clamps, favorite vibe, and butt plug along with a cane and crop in my nightstand, so that I can reach them from my bed. When the mood strikes, I don't want to be hunting around for what I want or need. Be prepared and make your bedroom—and your favorite sexy spots—easy to have sex in, whenever you desire. Just making space for sexual connection to happen will likely act as a catalyst for more intimacy and sex in your life.

Location, Location, Location

Let's set the scene for a romantic evening between you and your partner. What emotions does your bedroom currently evoke? Is it full of clutter and chaos? Baskets can be very helpful—sex baskets and kids' baskets. If you end up with a bunch of your kids' stuff in your bedroom that needs to be returned to its home, have a basket that you can throw everything into so you can return the items to their proper homes in the morning. Place "sex baskets" in the bedroom or even the bathroom if you find that you and your partner like to get intimate there. Decide what items assist you in that psychological shift from mama brain to sexy brain. What items turn you on? Is it a silk scarf or blindfold? The touch of a latex glove? Keep your sex basket stocked with what you need. Try to keep it out of reach of curious hands, and if your little one does get into your basket—and there is a chance that eventually this will happen—just explain that these are mommy's "non-sharing toys" and that it's okay to have things that are non-sharing items.

Taking sex out of the bedroom can be exciting too! Consider kitchen sex, bathroom sex, sex on the couch, or sex on the dining room table. Do you have a car? Or a garage or shed? A backyard where you can set up a tent? Bring the baby monitor and discover the sexual potential of locations surrounding your house, places where you can find the privacy and the refuge that your sexual self might be craving from the emotional responsibilities of parenthood.

Are you able to get a sitter for the night? Or have a friend or relative come over for an overnight? Getting a hotel room or an Airbnb and getting sexy in a different space can be a nice, decadent experience. Whereever you choose to go on your sexual adventure, the most important thing is to create space for connection and intimacy—whether that means holding hands, making out, or anal pleasure. Your sexual adventures can be packed with intimacy and emotion. Even if they only last a moment.

Make a moment last forever. As a parent, I have experienced so many fragmented intimate moments. And I've grown to love them all. When I first came into motherhood it was dreadfully frustrating. You're connected with your partner, he's looking into your eyes, he grabs your ass and pulls you in close to his body and leans in to kiss you—and then you hear "Mom! Can you come help me with wiping my butt? I need some help. It's a big poopy!"

Now I just laugh and transition seamlessly into the next moment of butt wiping, although part of me wishes we could just have marathon morning kitchen sex. But the intimate moments, they matter; they accumulate and they continue to fuel our connection, our love and desire for one another, and our ability to physically and emotionally connect and nourish one another. And so I learn to live and appreciate those moments. A hand running up his shirt to his fuzzy chest; his hand grabbing a fistful of my hair as he pulls me in close; his hand cupping my breast and clamping around my nipple; our intimate dance, chock-full of love and sometimes lasting less than a minute, providing us with a jolt of endorphins and a loving connection that fuels us for the rest of our day. I know I'm a better parent because of this nourishment, our connected moments. And I know our longer sexual romps and adventures have a greater depth due to the consistent nourishing moments of connection that we make with one another. The next time you kiss your partner, try to spill into that moment. Kiss with your entire body engaged. What are your arms and hands doing as you are kissing your partner? Your legs, your toes, your cunt? What is the distance between you and your partner while you kiss? Allow your kiss to be an opportunity to melt into one another and linger there for a moment.

REAL SHAG

Spicing up the bedroom as parents involves some degree of preparation and negotiation. REAL SHAG is a an acronym I use to remember what to review and discuss within BDSM scene negotiations, and this same acronym can be a helpful tool and reminder for parents about what they might want to manifest erotically between the sheets.

R: Roles—This is in reference to any role-play elements that you and your partner might want to take on as part of your sexual play, or any headspace that you might be wanting to explore, such as librarian and book lover, or soy milkman and vegan sex-starved soy milk–loving slut.

E: Expectations—If your partner says that he or she likes really rough sex or has always fantasized about being a sensation slut, well, those are very broad terms that can mean a lot of different things to different people. It's important for you to discuss how your partner actually envisions your sexual adventure and what his or her expectations are. Your partner should talk about specific sex acts or implements that he or she expects or envisions being used in your adventure, as well as the emotional tone of your experience. Is this an experience that you both want to keep light and playful? Slow and sensual? Or rough and aggressive—sex that really pushes one another's physical limits? Stating expectations and making sure that all partners are on the same page can assist in creating a sexual adventure in your bedroom—or beyond—that everyone enjoys.

A: Address—Whether or not you are exploring roles of dominance and submission, checking in about how each of you would like to be addressed during your adventure is key. You can be anyone you want to be. Remember, you can explore different roles and parts of your psyche as you step out of your parental roles and into your sexy self. You can take on another name. Another gender.

L: Length, Likes, and Limits—Knowing how long you expect your sexual adventure to last really helps in pacing yourself. Maybe the sitter is just at the park with your little one and they will be back in thirty minutes. And discussing your sexual likes and limits with your partner can help you both to draw a framework of boundaries and sculpt an adventure based on sexual acts and dynamics that really turn you both on. Even if you have been in a relationship with a partner for a decade or more, this can be helpful, as our desires, fantasies, and sexual likes/loves/limits are always changing and shifting.

S: Safe Words, Sexual Contact, and Safer Sex—Whether or not you and your partner are engaging in a kink scene or a vanilla adventure, safe words can be helpful to have. It's important to be aware of the vulnerability that both you and your partner engage in as you venture into new sexual adventures. Together you are exploring a new and intimate world. Let your partner know that if he or she needs to stop, he or she can say "Red" or "Yellow," and the two of you can stop and check in. We teach our children to use their words to state what they need, and we need to do the same. So use your words.

What type of sexual contact are you and your partner expecting? Maybe you are still sore and feeling anxious about vaginal penetration. Maybe your nipples are sore from breastfeeding. Maybe you have hemorrhoids from pregnancy, and the thought of anal pleasure sends shivers up your spine. These expectations, limits, and desires surrounding sexual contact should all be addressed between you and your partner prior to your sexual adventure.

Are you on birth control? Are you planning on using condoms? Knowing what type of safer sex methods you are using is important to spicing up your bedroom. Condoms can be super hot! Try putting a condom on with your mouth as part of your foreplay.

H: Health—Are there any health concerns that have come up during pregnancy or postpartum that you need to share with your partner? Check in with your body and make sure to communicate how it is feeling. Your sexual adventures don't have to include acrobatic porn-star sex positions or fucking upside-down from the chandelier. This is about sculpting a sexual adventure that fits your life and your body and enables you and your partner to connect in an intimate and pleasurable way.

A: Aftercare—*Aftercare* is terminology we use within the BDSM world to refer to the care of someone after a scene, and this pertains to all sexual adventures, really—especially when we are venturing into uncharted waters. Making sure you have a good support system set up for after a big sexual adventure can be really helpful. Communicating that might just mean something like this: "Honey, I'm having a lot of feelings about having sex for the first time since the baby, and I'm feeling kind of fragile. I think I'm going to need a warm bath and tea afterward, so if the baby wakes I'm going to need you to go in and rock her while I'm soaking for a bit." It's really about figuring out the care you might need when you go to a place that will involve a big endorphin rush, or a place that is really emotionally tender. I know for me there was a lot of emotional tenderness postpartum, and I found myself using an "emotional safe word" much more frequently and needing to be slow and gentle with myself.

G: Gear—What kind of gear will you need to bring for your sexual adventure? Any sex toys? Personal lubricant? Props? A water bottle? What elements does your sexual fantasy or sex basket require? You don't want to be fishing around the house for your flogger under a bunch of dirty laundry or rummaging through every drawer in the house to find a condom or lube when you finally have a moment alone with your sweetheart.

A SEXY MAMA'S POV
WITH CARLYLE JANSEN

After the birth of each of my children, I was not interested in sex at all. I was having a great time enjoying the connection with my kids and getting all of my feel-good feelings from the intimacy with them—which can actually be dangerous. Of course it is important to bond with our kids, and the physical connection that happens naturally for most of us can't be beat. But harmful patterns and expectations can emerge when we look to our relationships with our kids to fill all of our intimacy needs. It was important for me to separate out my adult needs and fulfill them though other connections.

As a single parent, I did not have an intimate partner right after each of the kids were born. So I had only myself to fulfill my sexual needs for several months. Dating was not on my radar, nor was sex. But I knew that it was important to keep those juices flowing and to have "adult" kinds of touch. I forced myself to get out my Hitachi Magic Wand on a regular basis to keep myself going even though I had no libido. Of course it always felt great and took very little effort, but I still had to force myself to make it happen. In the end it helped get me back in the game by keeping pleasure on my radar, getting my pelvic floor back into shape, and maintaining adult kinds of touch and response.

Now that I am partnered, it is still important to me that I have "adult time." I also believe that it is good for the kids to see that their parents have time to date and to nurture and prioritize their partnership. We plan outings on the town to continue having fun together and dating.

We also plan dates at home after the kids are in bed. They have a regular bedtime that they follow, which makes it easier for us to carve out an hour or two for ourselves. We still sometimes don't really feel like having sex, and it is not always on our radar, but we have learned how to initiate and get ourselves into a sexy headspace. (There are many times when we have planned a night in and start out by looking at each other awkwardly, knowing that sex is supposed to happen now.) Even when we are not planning sex, we devote some evenings to connecting on other levels. We have to be clear with each other that some nights are for connection; otherwise, our time together is spent on separate Facebook pages or doing our own work or play. We make a point of connecting intimately with a glass of wine or a foot massage, telling stories, talking about the relationship, or debating ideas so that we truly connect with each other—not just via text messages throughout the day about the kids, dog, and dinner.

Communication

WHAT ARE YOUR BOUNDARIES? How about your limits? What are your desires and fantasies? In our day-to-day getting by, it can be rare for us to find the time to examine these questions and find answers that we can use as a roadmap to following our desires and articulating our needs to our partners. The following exercises are a great catalyst for having this conversation with your partner. Try to let go of any preconceived ideas of what you think you might want or desire, and know that our desires ebb and flow throughout our lives, creating space for new explorations, new paths, new desires, and new limits based on what else is going on in our lives at the time. Let go of judgment and open yourself up to really listening and communicating with your partner about where you are today in your journey.

Negotiating Boundaries with Your Partner

Negotiating boundaries can be difficult. Many students at my workshops come to me and say that they have a really hard time communicating their limits to their partners. They are afraid that saying no or having boundaries and stating them will hurt their partner's feelings. So instead they say nothing. I have heard this same thing from women in their twenties, thirties, forties, and fifties. These women live most of their lives unable to honestly communicate their limits for fear of hurting their partners.

This is painful to hear, and it can feel absolutely dreadful to not have the words to communicate with your partner. Stating your boundaries and limits is just as important as stating your desires. It's true that sometimes we might not recognize a boundary until we have experienced it. But recognizing it and communicating about it with our partners can be incredibly healthy. Also, understanding our partner's boundaries and limits and respecting them is incredibly important. Knowing that our words are heard and honored and letting our partners know that their words are heard and honored is incredibly important as well. It further develops trust and space for intimacy and depth in our sexual lives.

Communicating your boundaries to your partner might look something like this:

"Honey, I love you and I love giving you fellatio, but I don't feel comfortable having sex in the same room as the baby. What do you think about having sex in the living room instead?"

Or:

"My love, I think your breasts are beautiful, and I think the fact that you are lactating is amazing, but I don't feel comfortable sucking on your breasts right now. Maybe that will change for me, but for right now that is a limit."

Or:

"Right now I'm feeling really sensitive about my belly and stretch marks. I'm still working on loving my body again and I think I need to reclaim that part of my body before I really have you touching me there. But I love your hands on my ass and breasts and in my mouth."

When stating a limit or boundary, it's helpful to give a little insight into the *why* of the limit, if you know (you might not), and give direction as to what you *do* want or desire. When you are doing this, you are not just saying *no,* but you are also saying *yes. No* to what doesn't work for you right now, and *yes* to what you want and need.

Remember the active listening skills we discussed in Chapter 7, and remember that you need to also listen to your partner about what feels good to him or her and what his or her boundaries are. When you hear something that you weren't expecting, that might feel disappointing. And you can state that: "Hmm. That's not what I was expecting. Sometimes it's difficult for me when things are different from what I expected, but I'm excited to try moving our lovemaking to the living room. Let me start to envision what that might be like."

Intimacy Exercise: Story Time

Story time is not just for the kids! Storytelling can be a great way of communicating with your partner and exploring your desires in a fun way that allows for listening and negotiation. In this exercise, you and your partner will tell a sexy story together. Sit down facing your partner and look into your partner's eyes, listening to your partner's words and following his or her story and journey. Hold space for your partner's fantasy to unfold. A story might begin like this: "Once upon a time, there was a woman who loved shoes. She really loved shoes. Not just to wear them, but to smell them and inhale the scent of leather that lingered in their innards."

After one minute of storytelling, the partner telling the story should let the other partner continue. I like to find ways to physically pass the story on, with a squeeze of the hand, a caress, or a kiss on the mouth. In your addition to the story, incorporate your own fantasies, but do *not* negate the fantasy world that your partner has just established. For example, in the example above, we discover that one partner has a shoe fetish. Here is an example of what *not* to do: "Although the woman thought she liked shoes, one day she woke up and decided that her fetish was really ridiculous and that cock was much better for sniffing than shoes."

Here is an example of how you could add your own fetish and fantasy to the story: "The woman walked into a shoe store and discovered a man hiding behind a curtain. She peered at him, his eyes meeting hers, and followed him behind the red velvet curtain into the dark warehouse. He beckoned to her with his fingers, and she crawled on her hands and knees past shelves and shelves of leather shoes, only to come face to boot with the tall mysterious man. She traced her way up his blue jeans and undid his leather-studded belt, grabbing his cock and engulfing it down her hungry slut throat."

I recommend five rotations of storytelling, or ten minutes total. At the end of the storytelling experience, each partner should take another minute to relate what he or she heard or discovered about the other partner, and then ask for clarification.

Here's an example of what this might look like: "What I think I'm hearing is that you are very turned on by shoes and that maybe you would be interested in further exploring a shoe fetish or shoe worship. Is that right? Can you tell me more?"

A SEXY MAMA'S POV
WITH SEARAH DEYSACH

Sex after having a kid is hard. And I'm not just talking about physically. In fact, I'm the non-birth parent in a two-mom household, so the physical aspect was a non-issue for me. Yes, my girlfriend, who carried our kid (thanks, honey!), had much body healing to do after birth, but the struggle to reintegrate sex back into our lives, even five years after our kid arrived, is also hard. We are tired and busy. Our kid is always around, and we still struggle with her sleep issues. So what is a couple to do?

We have come up with a few things that help keep the intimacy alive, if not the steamy hot sex of our pre-kid days. The most important part, I think, is letting each other know that we want to have sex, even if, for whatever reason, we cannot make it happen right now. When sex slows down, one can feel unwanted or unsexy, so telling your partner "Honey, your ass is so hot; I'd love to do you right now, but I have to get to the parents' council meeting" at least lets your love know he or she is wanted. Maybe add a slap on the butt or a sexy, deep kiss to hammer home your point. And then get to that meeting! I also like the idea of leaving a note for your partner, telling your partner what you would do to him or her if you had the time/energy/empty bed to make it happen. "I would love to bury my face between your thighs and pleasure you all night" is a good way to start.

I also think that one should never underestimate the power of masturbation to keep the sexy times going. If you are in the mood but your partner is not, try some solo play in your partner's vicinity. I know for a fact that having a partner getting off next to you is hard to ignore, and it very well might stir something in you that rouses you from your slumber enough to maybe at least lend them a hand (yes, that counts as sex!). Of course there are times when this is not appropriate or may annoy your partner, so know your audience, but sometimes we just need to be reminded that sex can be quick and easy to get our engines running.

Deep kissing is another way that I like to keep the romance alive. When you have kids, you might find you can go days without even properly greeting your partner, let alone showering them with love, affection, and sexy times. I actually put a reminder on my daily to-do list to make out with my lady so that I am reminded that we need, at the very least, a few seconds of intimacy per day. Those few seconds to refocus your attention on your sweetie, to remind yourself and your co-parent that you were once lovers, can go a long way toward helping you both feel loved, desired, and connected. And the bonus is that maybe it can lead to something a little more naughty.

18

Talking with Our Kids about Bodies, Gender, and Sexuality

THIS IS POSSIBLY ONE of the most challenging topics for many parents: How do we talk with our children about sex? *Do* we talk with our children about sex? If so, at what age, and how? Are we encouraging or pushing our children into adulthood or exploration of sex too early by giving them information? How do we possibly make "the sex talk" less awkward than the conversation we received from our parents—if we even received a single conversation about sex? These are just some of the many questions that I hear from parents regarding talking to their children about sex.

First I'd like for you to examine how you felt as a child about the way your parents talked about bodies and sexuality. Were you curious? Did you feel comfortable talking with your parents about your feelings? If not, what words or situations made you feel uncomfortable about asking your parents for the information you wanted? What worked for you and what didn't? How did that feel? What was helpful and what wasn't?

Exercise: Write a Letter to Your Child Self

Take a moment to write a letter to your child self. Answer the questions that you weren't able to find the answers to. Be compassionate and loving. Examine how you were feeling when issues of sex, gender, consent, and body image first arose in your life. What insight can you provide to your younger self now that you are an adult and have a child of your own?

Sex is a natural way in which humans connect and share intimacy and affection for one another. Sexual desire and sexual curiosity is perfectly normal. Learning about our bodies and their functions is empowering and helps a child to develop a sense of knowledge and agency surrounding their body. Teaching our children the power of "no" and empowering them with agency and consent surrounding touch and sharing of affection helps to build healthy communication around touch and body boundaries. Letting our children know that sex and gender are two separate things and that our genitals don't dictate someone's gender identity helps to empower children to make their own choices around gender expression and to avoid assuming someone's pronouns or gender identity without asking them. These are all skills that we can start to develop with our children from birth onward. The sex talk is not a single talk but an ongoing conversation with our children from the time that they are born. It exists in the way we handle questions like "What's this?" when our child spots our vibrator or a condom or lubricant or a tampon. It exists in our response when our infant reaches down for their genitals to pleasure themselves, and in the moment when we ask our child before giving them a kiss and respect them when they say no, because no means no. We teach our children how to ask for physical space by asking for it when we need it, and by noticing when our children need space and helping them to find the words to express what they need and to express their body boundaries. When we destigmatize sex and the expression of love and affection, the pursuit of pleasure, and our bodies, it makes conversing and answering questions about sex and the body so much easier.

When our children are nonverbal, we can still have a conversation about sex and bodies. This conversation is somewhat one-sided but your child is absorbing everything. For example, if your child does want to touch him- or herself, what is your reaction? Your child is simply engaging in touch that feels good. In the same way that massage or having your back scratched feels good, there is no shame in the experience. As your child grows into a toddler, you may want to set boundaries about self-touch. In our house, we tell our child, "It's a-okay to touch your vulva or anus, but we don't want to do that at the dinner table. If you would like some privacy for self-touch, you can do that in the bathroom or your bedroom." We also let our child know that she needs to wash her hands afterward. We explain that if we want to touch any of our mucous membranes, whether it's our vulva or mouth or inside of our nose, we need to wash our hands, because bacteria like moist areas and we need to keep our bacteria to ourselves so we don't get sick.

We can also start to develop concepts of consent and body knowledge with our children before they are verbal. One way in which we can start to impart these skills is by talking our baby through what we are doing. This is what it looks like: "I'm going to pick you up now, okay? All right, and now I'm just going to check to see if your diaper is wet. Yep, you are wet. Let's get you changed. I'm going to lay you down on the changing table now. There we go. Now let's get this diaper off of you and wipe off your vulva and anus and butt. There we go. All clean. Does that feel better?" With this language, we are letting our baby know what is going on and talking them through it as well as giving words and language for our child's body parts.

How to Talk with Your Kids about Consent

We've talked briefly about how to approach consent with our children when they are babies, but what about as they get older? As our babies grow into toddlers, we can practice consent with them through elements of play and with the touch that we give and receive. Are you playing with dolls or stuffed animals? Have the doll or stuffed animal ask your child for a hug: "May I have a hug?" If your child isn't super verbal, they can always nod or shake their head for *yes* or *no*. Have your child ask the stuffed animal or doll "Kiss?" in your play as well. The toy might respond, "I don't feel like a kiss right now, but I'd love a high five or a nose nuzzle." You can practice this same type of negotiation around touch between you and your child. Let your child know that if someone says *no* and doesn't want touch, that *no* always means *no* and that we respect body boundaries. One way to give affection when the other person isn't feeling like touch is to blow a kiss. Teaching how to negotiate touch and the many different ways to show physical affection arms your child with a very empowering skill. One of the ways we like to practice really listening to *no* is in tickling games or negotiated roughhousing. Our child loves to be tickled, and they are excellent about communicating where on their body they are comfortable being tickled. They will say, "Okay, I'm ready, tickle me!" which will result in massive giggles until I hear "Stop." *Stop* and *No* are both safe words and result in me immediately stopping and removing my hands from their body. Once they have recovered, they will say, "Go!" and we go for another round of tickling. We then switch places, and my little one will tickle me until I say "Stop." We always repeat the phrase "Stop means stop." On a regular basis, I remind my child that no one ever has a right to touch them without their consent. That it is their body and no one else's. I also remind them regularly—especially when they are really excited—to check in about body boundaries and touch before touching other people. When strangers touch my child—even a pat on the head—without asking, I see a flash of red in my child's eyes, and it's taken a while to work on a way to articulate that my child is not giving consent to this person to touch their body. Sometimes it is more of an eruption of "I did not give consent!" Which is true. The folks touching didn't mean any harm, but their touch is an invasion of my child's body and space. We have talked about taking a breath and getting a parent or teacher to help with the situation, or telling the person, "Excuse me. This is my body and I don't want my body touched unless I say so." It's a continued conversation as our children grow and become older. The key is planting those seeds and developing the conversation early on, and letting it develop over the years as your child's questions and communication develop.

How to Nurture a Healthy Relationship between Your Children and Their Bodies

Growing up, I was told not to look, talk about, or touch "down there." I didn't have any direction or education about what was happening to my body when I experienced menstruation, and I was fearful of my body. I didn't learn about my body or sexuality at home or in school, and I experienced deep shame surrounding my body and its functions. It took years to work through that shame and embrace my body, pleasure, and sexuality. Obliterating body and sexual shame became a huge emphasis and inspiration for my work as both an artist and sex educator, creating a deeper love of ourselves and others in the world. When I became a parent, I knew that above all, I wanted my child to grow up with a love and understanding of their body. Our sexual lives and the story of who we are really do start at birth. It doesn't determine who we will be, but it is a part of our journey, and I wanted my child's journey to start out from a place of love for themselves, their body, their vessel. This is our container for love. It's our shell. It's important to know how our bodies work and where we came from, and to have words for our body parts, not veils of shame and awkwardness.

The most basic thing I recommend is using anatomical names for your, your partner's, and your children's body parts and genitals. If you don't know the name for something, look it up. Female genitals should be referred to as the *vulva* (external) and *vagina* (internal); for a male, we say *penis* and *scrotum* and *testicles*. The bottom hole—where poop comes out—is the *anus*. Where does pee come out? The *urethra*.

When you change diapers or clothing, or during potty training or bath time—these are all great times to practice using proper language and names for body parts. Try not to say "ick" or "yuck" or "P.U." to butt wiping, diaper changes, accidents, or emptying the potty. By doing so, we associate our children's bodies with ickiness. It's natural. We all pee, we all poo—everything that eats pees and poos, and we are there for our children to help them navigate their bodies and their elimination process. It's a learning process, and we are their guides. When I started talking to my child about potty training and shifting from diapers to the potty, we started using training underwear instead of diapers, and when there were accidents, I'd say "It's uncomfortable when we go potty in our under-wear. It feels better for our bodies if we sit on the potty when we go pee and poop." I carried a little Ergo Potty with us everywhere we went, and at first we would set our timer and they'd sit on the potty every fifteen minutes. We'd have a huge celebration every time a pee or poo went into the potty. We would do a dance; we would sing; we would play with stickers and read books about going potty. Going potty was fun!

Way before we started potty training, I was still taking my child to the potty with me. Parenting coaches call this *graphic modeling,* but many parents will simply find that it's a necessity if you don't have another adult around to watch your little one while you go potty. So I'd talk about it. I'd narrate my actions: "Mommy really has to go pee-pee. Let's go to the potty. When mommy has to go pee-pee I sit on the potty. That feels much better. My pee-pee came out of my urethra and went into the potty and now I feel much better. Time to wash my hands. Mommy is taking care of her body and listening to her body." If I was menstruating, I would also get a chance to talk about menstruation: "This is mommy's menstrual cup. Once a month some of mommy's uterine lining breaks down and flows through my cervix, through my vagina, and into my menstrual cup." I'm able to speak more about this to my child the older they get.

There is no shame in being naked. Many children love to run around naked. Some adults do too. I wish I could run around naked more, but most of the time I'm freezing. My body runs cold, and my child's body is a warm heater. I'll be bundled up in a dozen layers while my child is running around in undies. However, when it is warm enough or when we are coming out of the shower, my child sees my body and my partner's body. We express our body boundaries around not touching: "My vulva is mine and not for you to touch. But if you feel like it, you can ask for privacy and explore your own vulva." Often I shower with my child, or we will take a bath together. We do not fear our bodies, and when my child has questions about my body, I answer them. Simply seeing other bodies around is a great catalyst for questions and conversations. We let our child know that clothing is something to keep our bodies warm and safe. If our child feels warm and wants to run around naked, that is totally fine. We ask that they carry a towel so that crumbs, dirt, and any gunk that didn't get swept up from their last art project doesn't end up in their vagina or anus.

We make art with bodies. My child has seen a lot of performance art, because I'm a performance artist. And my child loves making art. Often we make art with our bodies—paint with our feet, with our bellies, our butts, our hands. They also love to draw all over their body. This is a great way to know and love your body—seeing it as art, as sculpture, as a vessel for creative energy.

Make learning about your body fun! Our vulva puppet, Val the Vulva, made by House O'Chicks, has made conversations about bodies so much more fun. From conversations on anatomy to puppet theater renditions of "Mommy's Menstruating," Val the Vulva has come in handy many times in my parenting life. This anatomically correct vulva is beautiful and adorned with silk and sequins. Mine happens to be a genderqueer vulva with a Southern accent who uses the pronoun "they." We also have a cute egg and sperm stuffed animal set from the Giant Microbes collection. Make learning about bodies fun and accessible to your children. There are also great coloring books like Tee Corrine's vulva coloring book. And you can always get out a mirror. Many women who I meet in my workshops have never taken a good, long look at their vulvas. If your child is curious about his or her anatomy and wants to get a better look at the hole that poop comes out of or the hole pee comes out of or what her labia really look like, get out a small hand mirror and help your child to take a look at his or her body.

Age-Appropriate Answers to the Question "What is Sex?"

Cathy Winks, health educator and coauthor of *The Mother's Guide to Sex: Enjoying Your Sexuality through All Stages of Motherhood,* says it isn't really possible to give your child too much information. I agree that information is never a bad thing. Basically, if you give your kids more information than they are ready for, they will zone out or move on to another topic. When children are very young, they are mostly interested in basic concepts. Keep it basic and make sure that you know what question your child is asking, and answer that question instead of forging ahead with more information. You can say things like "People like to share touch and affection with one another. When we grow up to be adults, there are brand-new ways to share love and affection. Sex is one of the many ways that grownups can share affection and pleasure with each other." To a question like "What are you and daddy doing in the bedroom, and why is it so noisy?", you could say something like "Mommy and daddy are sharing grownup affection with one another. It's called *sex*. Sometimes I make a lot of noise because I get excited and it feels good for mommy's grown-up body." You could be even more basic in your explanation by saying, "We need space and privacy. Mommy and daddy are having special mommy/daddy time." Your conversation about sex and what mommy/daddy time means can grow as your child's questions grow. If you make sure not to shut down the conversation, your child will know that he or she can go to you and ask you questions when he or she has them.

What sex is *not:*

Sex is not just between a man and a woman. Let's not forget that individuals of any and all gender configurations can share adult affection with one another and experience pleasure together. You don't need to list every configuration; we're not trying to explain an orgy to a five-year-old here! Just take gender out of the equation: "Sex is shared, consenting adult expression of affection and pleasure between grownups."

Sex is not about love or marriage. We don't need to sing "The Birds and the Bees" along with the "Wedding March." Many people have children without getting married. My partner and I are still not legally married—though we are planning on getting married before this book is published. Just as kids don't pledge to be lifetime BFFs with every kid they hug or go on a play date with, grownups don't marry every person they have sex with. In fact, they might never choose to marry, and that is okay! That doesn't mean that they won't experience pleasure and find other adults to share grownup affection with. Sex is also not specific to love. Sometimes we feel like a hug, a massage, or a cuddle, and as adults, we might feel like sex. Just because it feels good doesn't mean that this action forever bonds us or equates to love. But it is a form of connection, affection, and mutual consenting pleasure.

Sex isn't just for making babies. In fact, I have never had sex in order to have a baby, but I have had a lot of sex, and one of those times resulted in a beautiful child whom I absolutely adore. Certain types of sex between an individual who has sperm and an individual who has eggs and a uterus can result in the creation of something that might one day develop into a baby. There are many ways to make a baby, and many children have different stories of how they came to their families. If you want to talk to your child about how babies are made, there is an excellent book that my little one loves called *What Makes a Baby?* by Cory Silverberg.

Forced touch is not sex. Touch that is forced and not negotiated or consented to is NOT SEX. Sex is always consenting. Non-consenting or forced touch, touch that violates one's desire not to be touched or that doesn't abide by "no means no," is not sex or shared affection of any kind. It's an act of violence.

Talking with Your Children about Safer Sex

If you and your partner use safer-sex supplies such as gloves, dental dams, or condoms, your child will likely point out a condom one day. Heck, even walking out in public, we have encountered discarded condoms. Perhaps your child will point to a package in the drugstore and ask what it is. So how do we start the conversation with our children about safer sex and safer-sex supplies that they might see in our bedrooms or out in the world? The way I like to present this to my child is that safer-sex supplies such as gloves, dental dams, and condoms go on body parts or objects that might enter or come into contact with blood or mucous membranes. The same gloves that are used in medical and dental offices can be used in the bedroom. These safety barriers help to keep bacteria or viruses that might be located in the blood or mucous membranes contained in one place. This is also why we don't really want to share cups, chapstick, lip gloss, or eye makeup. We can talk about these helpful barriers as a way to keep our bodies safe. Also, if you want to talk about condoms as birth control, you can explain how sometimes when people who have penises engage in grownup affection and get really excited, sperm exits their bodies through their penises. The condom keeps sperm in one place and catches it. This can also help to prevent sperm from meeting up with an egg in another person's body. I also let my child know that the condoms help to keep mommy's non-sharing vulva toys clean from bacteria from my anus, vulva, and vagina. Remember, when your children are really young, you simply need to meet questions with big-picture, confident, accurate answers that let them know that sex is a comfortable and safe topic to talk about.

Take Your Child's Lead

Listen openly and without judgment to what your child is asking, and if you don't have the answer or you need to think about how you would like to answer the question, let your child know: "That is a really great question. I'd love for us to talk about that later tonight." Pace yourself and start off with broad answers, providing more information if your child asks for details. Think about how you are really defining sex. Sex is much more than a physical act; it's a way in which grownups share affection and pleasure with one another. Make sure your child understands all the ways he or she can share affection: high fives, nose nuzzles, kisses, hugs, tickles, playful wrestling, blowing kisses, braiding hair, snuggling, dancing, and so many other ways. Sex is diverse too! It's just a form of sharing affection that works for grownup bodies and minds. It involves different kinds of touch between grownup bodies. There is an excellent series of books by Cory Silverberg that I *highly* recommend. The first book is called *Sex Is a Funny Word*. This comprehensive book is a thorough guide on how to talk with your children about sex.

Model Consent

When you are out with your friends and your child is there, ask your friends before hugging them. Model consent with your partner before kissing or crawling into your partner's lap. Our children are always watching, and we can't tell our children to ask for consent and then touch others without asking first or fail to stand up for our own body boundaries. Our everyday interactions with the world, and the ways we express our affection to our loved ones through touch, are all being absorbed by our children.

Teaching Children to Care for, Listen to, and Nurture Their Bodies

Caring for and knowing your body is all a part of body love and body positivity. This includes brushing teeth, brushing hair, and washing your belly, your toes, and your anus. We take care of our bodies and our hearts. Developing loving rituals, sharing a gentle meditation practice, or introducing yoga can all give your child practice in caring for his or her emotions, heart, spirit, and body. Learning to listen to their bodies and articulate their needs is a huge skill that your children will take with them as they learn more about their bodies and learn how to articulate their own desires, seek their own pleasure, and share affection with others.

Kids Might Explore Their Own Bodies, and That's Okay

It is perfectly normal for children to touch themselves. This may be something that you notice nearly from birth, or maybe it came up when your child was two or three years old. Maybe you haven't noticed this behavior in your child. The important thing is letting your children know that it is totally okay to touch their own bodies, and that it can feel very good sometimes. A good starting point is to let your children know where in the house they can have private space to explore their bodies— such as in their bedrooms or the bathroom—and that they need to wash their hands afterward. Establish safe space for your child's personal pleasure exploration as your child starts to explore and gets to know his or her own body.

State Your Own Body Boundaries and Encourage Your Child to Do the Same

Stating our own body boundaries is important in teaching our children how to state their body boundaries. If you don't want to have your child crawling on your body while you're on the phone, say to your child, "I see you want to be close to mommy. I have a body boundary right now that I don't want to have you on my lap. But I would love to have you close to me. Would you hold my hand, or would you like me to rub your back while I'm on the phone? Then we can have some lap time."

Gender versus Sex

Remember: Gender is between our ears; sex is between our legs. Gender and gender expression can be fluid or shift over time. Gender should not be assumed based on someone's appearance, and it's not determined by the genitals that someone might have. There are some excellent books for children that deal with gender and gender expression. Some of my favorites are *Morris Micklewhite and the Tangerine Dress, 10,000 Dresses, A Is for Activist, Rad American Women A–Z,* and *My Princess Boy.*

When I reference strangers out in public, I always use gender-neutral pronouns and refer to the person as a person, not a woman or man. We don't know how that person identifies, and we can teach our children not to gender people by identifying and valuing them as individuals and not identifying them as a certain gender. Let's challenge our very gendered society and create some space for our children to find their own gender expressions, not fight their way out of gender expressions that have been imposed on them.

We are raising a new generation of sex-positive, body-positive children who are developing their emotional toolboxes early on and creating a solid foundation for consent and the exchange of love and affection. We are teaching them a positive view of sex and their bodies, armed with knowledge and the know-how to ask when they don't know the answers. Our children are a part of the next generation, and together, through educating and serving as a resource and guide for them, we will help them become a generation that doesn't hide from sexual conversation in fear or shame, but accepts as a natural part of our human experience the seeking of pleasure and connection with other individuals.

A SEXY MAMA'S POV
WITH LUCKY TOMASZEK

My children are barely children any longer. I am now the nearly middle-aged mother of three young adults. They are really decent human beings, and I'm proud of them. When my oldest daughter was approaching adolescence, I had frequent flashbacks to the power struggles of my youth. Memories of vicious arguments with my own mother haunted me, and I wanted desperately to walk a different path with my kids. I asked myself: What would have made that relationship better? I came up with two things that would have helped me back in the day, and I turned them into the philosophies that guided the way I parented my teens.

The first was something my older sister said to me when I was a young adult living on my own and really struggling to get on my feet. After a very frustrating day, she wrapped me up in a warm hug and whispered, "Your side is the only one I care about." Those words meant that someone really saw me and wanted the best for me. I have said this very thing to my teenagers so many times now. They know it's true, and it helps them feel comfortable bringing me their stories. It doesn't mean that I never help them correct course, nor does it mean that they always get a pass for bad behavior. But it does mean that I will strive to understand their motivations and help them through the rough stuff.

The second thing was born from my experiences as a teenager. I didn't get my driver's license until my twentieth birthday. My mom was a single parent, often exhausted by long working hours and the stress of doing everything by herself. Unexpected requests for rides often created resentment that could last for a couple of days. As a result, I spent a lot of my teenage years feeling stranded, sometimes in bad and dangerous situations. When I reflected on this as an adult, I realized that teenage me wanted to be able to call mom for a ride, anytime, for any reason. So my second tenet for parenting my teens has been, "I will always come for you."

My kids have tested me in big ways on this a few times, but I have never faltered. (They have also never abused it, which helps a lot.) This philosophy means that I get interrupted in the middle of dates and in the middle of sleeping. It means that sometimes I walk away from an unfinished meal or have to leave work unexpectedly. None of that matters. When I've retrieved one of them from a sticky situation, and they're pouring their heart out on the drive home, I know it's the right thing. They tell me the whole story, ask for feedback, and seek safety in our family home.

Living this way means not only that my kids trust me, but also that I can trust them. Even when it comes to sex. We have frank conversations about consent, contraception, STI prevention, sexual pleasure, gender identities, sexual orientation, and more. These topics are woven honestly into our everyday communication. I've never needed to set aside time to have "the talk" about any of this. It has all just come authentically from living a life where my kids know they can count on me, and I know they'll come to me when they need to.

A SEXY MAMA'S POV
WITH MADISON YOUNG

When I found out that I was pregnant, I knew I was birthing a revolution—a change deep inside myself that would alter my world forever. I knew that if I was going to be a parent, I would parent as a feminist. Parenting was political, the ultimate radical relationship. A foundational relationship of firsts.

As parents, we are a child's first experience in developing and experiencing love and intimacy. We hold space and guide our little ones as they develop a relationship to their bodies and to the bodies close to them. With an emotional coach by their side, they learn how to articulate and express their feelings and what they want and how to give affection using their words. They learn the meaning of "no" and the importance of consent.

Until I was really in the thick of parenting, I had no idea how all of these concepts and my feminist practices would come into play in the real world. But in the grand tradition of DIY, I am learning by doing, by connecting, by communicating, by listening and creating space for authentic expression of self.

Em is what you call a spirited child, chock-full of emotions and creative visions. I didn't get the quiet, chill Buddha baby—I got a unique child who challenges me in every way. A kid who came out kicking and screaming with an "I am here!" personality that doesn't go unseen or unheard. I don't think that I really could have expected anything less.

Here are some of the radical lessons I've learned along the way, and some of the challenges and successes I have met with in my adventures of raising a feminist.

Gender Expression

I gave my child the name Emma, after the radical feminist anarchist Emma Goldman, whose fiery words had inspired me in my work as an artist and activist. By the time my child was two years old, they were expressing a desire to identify as neither girl nor boy. Their name shifted and changed from Emma to Emmerson to Em to Femme. Their gender and pronouns bounced from "he" to "she" to "they," ebbing and flowing as their vocabulary and expression of gender widened and became more complex.

This was not unusual for me. As a queer mama, I made sure to have a full library of gender-diverse books for Em. I mindfully avoided gendering the characters in fairy tales or the people around us. For example, if we saw a person walking down the sidewalk, I wouldn't identify that person by perceived gender but would instead say something like "Do you see that person across the street in the bright yellow raincoat? I wonder if they think it will rain." I taught Em not to make assumptions about people's pronouns or genders and to ask what someone's preferred pronoun was.

I would check in with Em on a daily basis: "Hey darlin', what's your preferred name and pronoun today?" Em would inform me of their choices, and that was that.

Kids at the playground would ask, "Hey! Hey! Is that a boy or a girl?"

I would respond with "You will have to ask them."

"Hey! Hey! Are you a boy or a girl?" the kid would ask Em.

"I'm not a boy or a girl, I'm just a kid" was generally Em's response.

Sometimes the kids on the playground would be

frustrated by this response. "Don't they know if they are a boy or a girl?" "They can't be both." "They don't get to choose." These were some of the responses that I heard. But Em was choosing and letting us know, and we listened.

Consent

"I wanna hug dolly. Em hug dolly," Em demands at one and a half.

"Ask the dolly if the dolly wants a hug," I suggest.

"Dolly hug?" Em asks, reaching out for the dolly.

I pick up the dolly and respond, "I don't feel like a hug, but I'd love a big kiss."

"Big KISS!" Em claps her hands, happy with the type of intimacy that they and dolly have negotiated.

Em is two and chasing a cat. I call Em over to me and have them sit on my lap. "Em, do you think the cat wants to be touched right now?"

"I don't know," Em mumbles, looking at their shoes.

"What is the cat doing with its body?" I ask.

"Playing tag." Em smiles.

"Cats can't consent to touch with words, so we need to listen to their body language. If you present your hand when you're still and calm with your body and the cat comes over and rubs up against your hand, then it is saying yes to some gentle touch. If it runs away, it is saying, 'Space please.'"

Em is four years old. "I want ticka bugs!" they say.

"Okay. Here they come. Ticka bugs are coming!" I say as I tickle Em's belly and ribs.

They roll around on their mattress, laughing and wriggling under my touch. "Stop. Stop," they say breathlessly *in a burst of laughter, and my hands stop immediately and return to my own body.*

"Stop means stop," I say, reminding Em of our safe word. "Whenever we say stop, it's always important to stop our bodies right away, right?" I confirm, making sure that I can see Em's eyes, so that I know Em is focused and listening.

"Right!" Em says. "Now go!" they exclaim with robust enthusiasm.

I continue our tickling game, and then Em asks, "Can I tickling you, mama?"

"Yep. But only on my belly, not on my feet, okay?" I say, stating my desired tickle touch for our physical play.

"Okay dude-a-rama!" Em yelps in excitement as they leap into tickling.

"Stop, stop," I laugh.

Em stops their hands. "Stop means stop."

"Go!" I say, and our physical display of affection and connection continues as we respect one another's words and limits.

When we go to a park, the mall, the market, sometimes a person standing beside us will look at Em and smile, then pet Em's head. There is nothing that Em despises more, and every time, this touch is met with a deep belly roar and a grumble—often followed with a loud voice screaming, "I did not give CONSENT!"

We are currently working on gentler ways of communicating about unwanted touch from strangers, such as "I don't like it when you touch my head. Please stop." But I do think that Em's current response is closer to what their namesake Emma Goldman would belt out.

Body Acceptance and Body Love

Em loves to run around naked. Em is a spirited child. Did I mention that already? This spirited kid is always warm, even when others are chilly. Em is also really sensitive to textures and materials, so running around in the buff as much as possible is Em's thing.

Em loves their body and loves to play the drums with their round belly. They will spend an hour making belly prints or using their entire body to paint with finger paints. We let Em know that clothes are for protecting our bodies, keeping us warm when we feel cold and keeping dirt and bacteria out of our orifices and mucous membranes. When Em wants to run around naked, I just have a rule that they need to put a towel down to protect their body.

Body Knowledge

"Head, shoulders, uterus and vulva, uterus and vulva," my two-year-old and I sing as we identify the parts of our body. Growing up, I didn't have a word for my genitals; my mother, who works in the medical profession, wouldn't give my vulva or anus a name. My genitals were referred to as "down there" and "unmentionables" and "your you-know-what". But the problem was, I didn't know what, and it was really disempowering. This lack of knowledge fueled my tiny body with a lot of shame and fear around my body parts. My parent's body shame reinforced a really unstable relationship with my own body. And it took years to reclaim and smash that stigma.

That absence of a foundational education fueled my career in sex education and inspired me as an artist to further the conversation of body awareness. Obliterating the stigma surrounding sex became a primary goal of my artistic practice. In removing this stigma, I believe that we have the ability to advocate for healthy relationships with our own bodies and to navigate healthy sexual relationships with others.

So how do I counter that as a mom? Em receives the knowledge that they seek as a curious four-year-old child. Em has names for their body parts, and they learn more about their own body as they continue to develop and ask more detailed questions and I provide age-appropriate answers.

We use language like vulva and anus to describe our anatomy, and Em knows the ins and outs of menstruation. Em can answer questions such as "What is menstruation?" "Why do some people menstruate?" "When do some people menstruate?" "What does menstrual blood look like?" In fact, I think Em knows more about menstruation than I did when I first started to menstruate at twelve years old. Em understands that every month my body releases an egg, and that the egg journeys from the ovaries to the fallopian tubes to the uterus and out the tiny hole of the cervix and comes out of the vagina along with some shedding of the walls of the uterus.

Em has a coloring book of vulvas, and they decorate diagrams of the uterus with purple glitter and watercolor paints. We have lively puppet shows on the topic of body awareness with our plush toy egg and sperm and our genderqueer vulva puppet, Val the Vulva.

We discuss what is healthy for our bodies and what isn't healthy for our bodies—not what is right and what is wrong. We do talk about what is gentle and not gentle. We have frequent talks about the importance of consent, body *agency, and ways to communicate with others about the type of affection we would like to give.*

Em knows that no one has a right to touch any part of their body without consent. It is okay for Em to explore the touch of their own body and what feels good to them, but until both people are grownups, any giving or receiving of touch around mucous membranes is inappropriate. This includes kids sticking their fingers in each other's noses or mouths. Em understands what mucous membranes are, and they get that these are areas that have bacteria that are unique to each person's body, and that we don't want to share that bacteria with others.

If Em chooses to explore touch of their mucous membranes in a private area like the bedroom or bathroom, that is totally okay. They just ask, "Privacy, please," and wash their hands afterward.

I keep a box of nitrile gloves by the bedside table, and Em noticed that these are the same type of gloves that they see at the doctor's office and the dentist's office. When Em asked me why I had "doctor gloves" in the bedroom, I was able to explain that they acted as a barrier for bodies when entering a mucous membrane area. A few months later, Em found a condom—still in the package—and inquired about it. I took a breath and was able to make what could have been an awkward situation totally normal and to take the power and stigma out of a conversation about condoms. Because we have already had conversations about bodies, mucous membranes, and barriers, I was able to explain that the condom is a barrier for mommy's non-sharing vulva toys or a grownup penis or a hand that might come in contact with a mucous membrane. Body knowledge is power.

There Is No Wrong Section of the Toy Store

I love my father. I do. But we have different ideas around gender roles. When we went back to Ohio this past Christmas to visit the family, grandpa wanted to take Em shopping for toys. Em put a doll in the cart first, and then headed towards the yellow Tonka dump trucks. Em had it on their Christmas list, along with a spaceship and a Matchbox race car set.

As Em sprinted toward the trucks and race cars, they heard those words for the first time: "I think you're headed to the wrong section of the toy store, young lady," grandpa said. Em's heart sank; their mouth hung open and they stared at grandpa with the truck in hand. I dove in toward Em. "There are no wrong sections of the toy store, grandpa," I said. "These toys are for everyone."

Sharing the Mic

As an artist, author, and filmmaker, I travel and tour frequently for work, and sometimes I'm able to include Em on those tours. It's both an exhausting and a rewarding experience to tour with my little one. There is not really any downtime when you're touring with a kid. When you're not working, you're "on" as a parent.

Em has been traveling internationally with me for tours since they were a baby, so they adapt fairly well while on tour, which often involves new sitters, new foods, trains, planes, boats, and long days. It's work, and it's a lot of transitions for a kid.

Em knows when I'm working on my writing or an art exhibit and will say that they have work to do too. Em will fill up multiple journals and sketchbooks with pen and ink drawings of how they see the world as we are traveling.

When we came across an anarchist library during a recent tour in Sydney, Australia, Em was eager to explore the library, as was I.

Em assertively went to the counter and shouted, "'Scuse me! 'Scuse me!" at a man covered in tattoos and dressed in all black, staring at a computer.

The gentleman looked down and found Em looking up at him. He was a bit surprised. "Yes?" he asked.

"Where's your kids' section?" Em asked.

"Hmm. We don't have a kids' section, but I have a few things you might like." He brought a cardboard box down from a high shelf, and Em's eyes widened as they spotted a guitar.

Em plucked the guitar from the box and immediately jumped into the window seat in front of the store full of punks and anarchists. I smiled. It was my turn to sit back and let Em have the mic.

Em looked out at the small audience. "Would you like to hear something light or something dark?" Em asked them.

"Play some Slayer, kid!" a young teenager shouted with laughter.

Em looked up, shooting her a glare, and responded with "I'll just play something that is light and dark."

I tapped the young lady on the shoulder and whispered with a smile, "They only play originals."

Em proceeded to play for a good fifteen minutes, which is a pretty impressive set of original material for a four-year-old! I was thoroughly impressed.

CHAPTER

19

Toys

IF YOU ARE ALREADY a mom, you might find that you spend way
too much of your time picking up your kids' toys from the chaotic storm
of playdates and glittery art projects in your home. But don't forget that
your children are not the only ones who can enjoy toys! Mommy needs
time to play too, and it doesn't hurt to update your toy box with some
new treasures, whether you are an expectant mother or a mom of three.
So let's take a look at some toys and techniques that can make both solo
mommy time and play dates with your partner much more fun.

All of the following techniques and advice are given with the assump-
tion that you are experiencing a pregnancy that is free of complications
and that you haven't been advised otherwise by your physician regarding
penetration, sex, or orgasm. Make sure that you have a physician who
you feel comfortable talking to about sex and what is okay for your
specific pregnancy. Each pregnancy is different. Remember, there are
so many ways to express and explore your sexuality and sexual pleasure
with your partner.

Using Toys during Pregnancy

As long as your physician hasn't advised otherwise, toys in general
are perfectly okay to use during your pregnancy. As your pregnancy

progresses, your cervix will thin, and in general you don't want to be too rough on your cervix, as it could cause some bleeding. That said, dildos, strap-ons, and vibrators can all be great fun during pregnancy. I found that my pregnancy was a very juicy and orgasmic nine months for me. I was raging with hormones and horny all the time. I masturbated constantly and ejaculated more than ever! I was inseparable from my Hitachi Magic Wand and my Mystic Wand throughout my pregnancy. I did quite a bit of international travel, so my battery-operated Mystic Wand ended up being quite handy as an alternative to an electric-powered vibe that would require a power converter. Check in with your body during your pregnancy and see what sensations you might be craving. Before my pregnancy, soft, sensual touch had very little impact for me. I had always found light touch and sensation to be more annoying than anything, but during my pregnancy, soft, sensual, luxurious touch felt decadent and delicious! Silk scarves, feathers, massage oil, warm wax, the hug of silk and cashmere rope around my chest, and the light squeeze of tweezer clamps as opposed to my clover clamps—it was so erotic! Long, full-body sessions of making out and massaging my legs and vulva with oils felt magical, and strap-on sex with a light vibe on my cunt brought me to some of the most ecstatic, mind-altering places that I've ever experienced. I also really enjoyed anal pleasure throughout my entire pregnancy, both manually and with anal plugs and my Lucite dildo. Many women experience hemorrhoids during pregnancy, but I didn't have that problem and was able to enjoy anal pleasure throughout pregnancy. Everyone's body is different, so listen to your body and indulge in the toys and activities that call to you.

Using Toys during Labor

I don't know why it wasn't mentioned in *What to Expect When You're Expecting,* but vibrators are an incredible pain-relieving tool during labor. I labored using several of my toys. During the first twelve hours or so I used my Hitachi Magic Wand. The Magic Wand had gotten me through many a painful S&M scene in my past, and indeed, it did make the first day of my labor more orgasmic and sent lots of yummy endorphins through my body as my cervix began to open with each contraction.

Later in my laboring process, I opted to get into a birthing tub. It was so soothing, and I used the waterproof Mystic Wand in the tub during the latter part of my laboring. Again, it served as a welcome sensation to my body, vibrating goodness while my body felt as if it were splitting in two.

Using Toys Postpartum

During my postpartum experience, I was so sore! My erotic center shifted from my cunt and anus to my mouth in those first couple of months after giving birth. I felt uncertain about my body below my shoulders—*What is happening with my breasts? My cunt is so swollen! My belly is so tiger-striped!* It took me a while to embrace these parts of myself again, but my mouth—my mouth was the same sexy, pillowy red lips that I knew and loved! I knew how to give affection with my mouth, and it was something that was a pleasure not only for the person receiving, but for me. I loved giving my partner blow jobs or performing analingus, or suckling on a female partner's breasts. But I also loved masturbating by gently massaging my vulva and orally pleasuring my VixSkin dildo. It felt so good in my mouth. This was also a great dildo for me as I started to play with penetrative toys again, because the VixSkin dildo's silicone skin is soft and gentle. Kegelcisers such as Betty Dodson's Vaginal Barbell and the Smartballs by Fun Factory were a big help once I was approved for penetration again. These Kegel-focused toys helped me build the strength of my PC muscles back up after the birth of my child. As I was able to build PC strength, the strength of my orgasms built up again, and I was able to gain greater strength and build my erotic power by the simple tightening and flexing of my PC muscles.

Using Toys throughout Motherhood

There are so many sex toys out there to explore! And a mother's toy box need not have any limits. I highly advise ordering toys from women-owned, feminist, or sex-positive toy stores, rather than going to dimly lit sex shops where the clerks are not well educated about their products. Find a toy store that resonates with your politics, one where you can receive direction from sales associates who are also educators and have a greater knowledge of the body and sexual pleasure and health. You want to make sure that you are buying toys that are healthy to have in your body. Many of the cheaply made toys are made with chemicals that act as irritants to our bodies. Look for toys that are BPA free, phthalate free, and nonporous. If your toy is porous, that means that when you introduce it to your body, bacteria from your body can become trapped in the toy. Bacterial growth in your toys can result in the spread of bacterial infections. Most sex-positive toy stores, such as goodvibes.com and babeland.com, will almost exclusively offer nonporous and BPA free toys. But always check. Some toy materials that are BPA free and nonporous include silicone (including medical-grade silicone), stainless steel, glass, and Lucite. If the box you are looking at does not say BPA free and nonporous, then it is likely not BPA free. If you are able to smell the toy, does it have a strong chemical smell? If you are absolutely in love with an element of a toy that does have a chemical smell and you are questioning its material composition, but you still want to try it out, you can try using it with a condom. If you use one of these toys without a condom, you will likely experience a burning sensation. This is your body telling you that you shouldn't be sticking chemical-filled toys in your mucous membranes! So if you have a question about a toy's composition, put a condom on it. Otherwise, purchase only high-quality toys that are healthy for your body.

While we are on the subject of what is healthy for our bodies, let's talk about lubricant. After giving birth, you might notice a lack of lubrication in your vagina. This is due to a hormonal shift that occurs postpartum. Even when I was sopping wet during pregnancy, I still enjoyed adding even more lubricant to my vulva and vagina. Lubricant just makes everything even more slick and moist and slippery. There is no shame in using lubricant. It's not only for folks who can't produce enough of their own. I have heard people say things like, "Oh, my girlfriend doesn't need lubricant. I can get her plenty wet." Even if you can produce loads of natural lubricant, depending on how long you are experiencing penetration or the type of sex you are having, adding additional lubricant can just feel good. It's that simple. But finding the right lubricant is a personal choice, and finding one that you really like can really feel wonderful and empowering and make you want to engage in sexy times even more often. If you give someone a massage, you would apply lotion or oil to increase the pleasure of the massage, right? Lubricant ups the sensation and pleasure factor for sexual intimacy in a similar way.

Many drugstore brands of lubricant contain glycerin, which is a sugar compound. You might notice that lubricant with glycerin has kind of a sticky, tacky quality to it. If you rub this glycerin-based lubricant between your thumb and first two fingers and then pull your fingers apart, you might see some webbing from the lubricant. It has a gummy quality. If used for vaginal penetration, it can also encourage the growth of yeast and increase the risk of yeast infections. So I encourage you to watch out for this ingredient and avoid it.

You can find numerous types of lubricants on the market, which fall into three main categories.

Water-based lubricant—This type of lubricant is water soluble. The most widely used and available lubricants are water based. This is also the type of lubricant in which you are most likely to find glycerin, so be cautious when purchasing water based. There are some great, gentle water-based lubricants, but you really need to do your research on ingredients. Water-based lubricant is also absorbed into the skin during use, so this type of lubricant generally requires you to continue to reapply. If you're planning on having sex in the water, this is likely not a good fit for you, as it will dissolve. There are several types of water-based lubricants. The two most common types are a gel-like texture that tends to be more viscous, and a cream-like texture which is thin and similar to lotion. Water-based lubricants are safe for use on sex toys, and are compatible with safer-sex materials such as condoms, gloves, and dental dams.

Silicone lubricant—This is typically my favorite type of lubricant. Most silicone lubricants are latex safe, so they are compatible with safer-sex materials. The cool thing about this lubricant is that it is glycerin free and is not absorbed into the body by our skin or our mucous membranes! Because of this, silicone lubricants last longer than water-based lubricants, and are also effective when having sex in the water. But it's slippery stuff (don't slip in the tub!) and can be difficult to get out of the sheets—so be careful. The slippery texture and silky smoothness of silicone lubricant is a big turn-on for me. If you do plan on using this type of lubricant with any of your silicone toys, make sure to use a condom on your toy, as silicone will bond to itself; this can change the texture of your toy, which creates a tacky or sticky texture and also compromises the material, causing breakage which could harbor bacteria.

Natural oil–based lubricants—Oil-based lubricants can compromise latex safer-sex supplies and cause breakage of condoms during use. Oil-based lubricant is really best if you are with a partner to whom you are fluid-bonded and not using condoms, or if you are using a toy that doesn't require a condom. My favorite oil-based lubricant is coconut oil. This can have a nice slippery feel to it, minus the glycerin that you find in many water-based lubricants. It's also nice that it is all natural! Coconut oil is absorbed by the body, though, so it does require reapplication. And it comes in solid form, so you need to rub it between your hands first to liquefy it before applying it. I keep a jar by my bed for personal use and a jar in the kitchen for cooking!

The sex-toy industry has grown exponentially over the past decade, and the types of toys vary as widely as the individuals that use them. You can find eco-friendly solar-powered vibrators; vibrators powered by your USB; dildos made from stainless steel (Njoy), twenty-four karat gold (Jimmy-Jane), or medical-grade silicone (Fun Factory and Lelo); hand-blown glass toys (Fucking Sculptures); and even beautiful wooden sculpted sex toys that are coated in a nonporous polymer coating (NobEssence). There is something for every mama! Here are a few options to get you started.

Vibrators—Vibrators are sex toys that...vibrate! They come in every shape and size imaginable. There are external vibrators—such as the Hitachi Magic Wand or Mystic Wand—and there are also insertable vibrators that you can use both externally and internally for vibration during penetration. Vibrators can be a blast to use by yourself or with your partner. They don't have to be just for solo play. It can be so fun to have your partner tease you with a vibrator or put a small vibe on your clitoris while you are being penetrated, or to give your partner the remote control to a remote-controlled vibe for a really fun evening! You'll find that some vibrators and sex toys have a curve to them. These toys can be a lot of fun to play with if you are interested in stimulating your G-spot! The G-spot is one of many erogenous zones on female-bodied individuals. It's a glandular tissue that surrounds the urethra; it's also referred to as the paraurethral sponge. It's located on the ceiling of the vagina, about two inches in. Toys or fingers that are pointed upward, toward the belly button, will stimulate the paraurethral sponge. This can be arousing for many individuals, but generally, it feels better if it's stimulated once you're already aroused. So don't go straight for the G-spot—advise your partner to engage in some foreplay first and really get you hot before searching for it. The more aroused you are, the larger your G-spot will become, because the G-spot is a glandular tissue—which means that as you become more aroused, it starts to fill with a glandular fluid (ejaculate). So it will be much easier to find once it's really aroused and swollen. The paraurethral sponge is textured—it feels kind of ruffled or ridged. It's easiest to find it with your fingers first, and then introduce well-lubricated, curved toys. Generally, a firm touch is ideal for stimulating the G-spot, but experiment and see what feels good to you. Try it out yourself first and then guide your partner through G-spot play. I often enjoy continued clitoral or external stimulation while experiencing direct G-spot stimulation. If you feel as if you have to pee when engaging in this type of sexual play, it's because your G-spot is full of that glandular fluid. We release the fluid by pushing outward with our PC muscles. The fluid will exit from your paraurethral sponge through your urethra, which is why you might first feel like you have to pee. But although both exit through the urethra, urine empties from our bladder, while ejaculate empties from the glandular tissue. I wasn't able to ejaculate right after giving birth. In fact, it took about a year and a half after I gave birth to strengthen my PC muscles and relax into my body enough to release my ejaculate. I had incredible sexual experiences and orgasms, but my ejaculation went on a dry spell postpartum. All of our bodies are different, so know that wherever you are on your sexual journey, you can lean into pleasure, relax, and ease up on expectations. We are always changing, and your body will continue to evolve on this sexual journey as you journey onward.

If you do find yourself wetting the sheets with gushes of ejaculate, waterproof bedding can be a great way to protect your mattress. Also, hospital-grade cloth Chux pads can be super helpful to have next to the bed for easy cleanup.

Incognito sex toys—Whether you choose to have a locked treasure chest full of mommy's non-sharing vulva toys, have your toys out in the open, or perhaps opt for a little more discretion, incognito sex toys can be fun! It can also just feel really sexy to have your vibe or sex toy with you in your makeup case or purse disguised as a lipstick, or dangling around your neck while you're at the PTA meeting. My favorite is the Crave clitoral stimulator that doubles as a fashionable silver pendant. It charges via USB and I wear it almost every day. These toys can also add convenience—for example, the I Rub My Duckie is a waterproof vibe shaped like a rubber duck. It can live in your shower for whenever you want to have a quickie after your wee one is in bed.

Anal plugs—Oh, the joys of anal pleasure! I'm not going to lie: I love anal play. I loved it before becoming a mom and I love it after becoming a mom. It is important to remember a few key things when engaging in anal pleasure:

1. Relax. If your anus is tight and clenched, it will not be receptive to touch, sensation, or pleasure.

2. Take your time. Your anus might need some warm-up. Have your partner massage the backs of your thighs and your butt cheeks, gradually moving closer to your anus during the massage. Apply lots of lubricant and spend plenty of time just massaging the anus—all external. We are relaxing the anus and letting it know that it is okay to relax and to receive pleasure. Massage the anus with small circles and apply a little pressure. After lots of lube and external massage, press a toy (or finger or thumb) against the anus and wait for the anus to relax, start to open, and suck in the toy. Fingers are a great way to warm up before presenting a toy. Be sure to continually add lubricant— your rectum does not produce its own lubricant, and the anal walls can easily tear if you're not careful. I always prefer silicone lubricant for anal stimulation.

Also, when selecting a toy, make sure that the toy you choose has a flanged or flared bottom. Although the vagina is a cul-de-sac, the rectum is not. Safety first, mamas!

There are so many fun anal plugs out there—anal plugs that vibrate, anal plugs that you can leave in while you go out on a date—HOT!—and even jeweled anal plugs! What does your partner think about anal pleasure? Everyone has an anus—no matter what gender—and exploring the erogenous zones and tissue around the anus and rectum can be a whole new sexual adventure for you and your partner.

Strap-ons—Anyone can strap it on, whether you have a cock or not. You can be a sexy mama with a strap-on that your partner pleasures with his or her mouth, anus, breasts, or cunt. Your partner can strap on a dildo with a traditional harness that goes over the vulva or cock, or he or she can strap on a thigh harness or two! You can create your own multi-cock fantasy with only one partner and multiple strap-ons. As a woman, I've also found that it can feel incredibly hot to strap on a cock, slip a small vibe into the strap-on, and jack off my silicone strap-on cock as I massage and press the base of the cock up against my vulva. Experiment with a new way of masturbating and expressing your gender or sexuality.

Whether your style is satin with pink leather and glitter or butch with masculine biker studs, there is a strap-on out there for every shape, size, and expression of self.

CHAPTER

20

Oral

I KNOW THERE ARE times when we are so radically exhausted from parenting that sex is the last thing on our minds. If we can't find time to put food in our mouths and feed our bodies, how will we ever find time or motivation to fill our mouths with our partners' bodies and feed our sexual needs?

First of all, relax. We are all exhausted, and parenting can be exhausting—especially on top of work, household management, and basic self-care. Our energy, sleep, and even sexual desires and needs will ebb and flow. What helps is if we can take an assessment of where our energy levels and sexual desire are at this moment in time, and find a place of love and acceptance for our bodies and our desires and capabilities that exist in that moment. Our partners' energies and sexual needs will ebb and flow as well, but not always at the same time as ours. And although we might be exhausted, intimacy and touch can be nourishing. If you are feeling exhausted, find ways to explore intimacy within that state of exhaustion.

Want to jump-start your libido? Try lying next to your partner and clenching and releasing your PC muscles (doing your Kegels). As you are tightening and flexing these muscles, visualize calling forth your partner's body with just your PC muscles. Imagine a rope tethered to your partner;

you are pulling your partner closer to you using the strength and desire between your legs. Start to incorporate your breath into your exercise, drawing forth your partner and tightening your PC muscles with your inhale and releasing your PC muscles and your desire with your exhale. You can also rock back and forth or make small pelvic circles. Draw your partner close using your movement, energy, and breath, and then release and bring a mindfulness to your erotic energy. Feel its power and visualize its color and texture as it embraces you both.

Certain sexual activities take more energy than others. And sexual techniques can take on a variety of expressions. The blow jobs or cunnilingus that you give or receive don't always need to be a fast, hardcore, raging punk song. Explore the slow sensuality of a slow dance and amp up the intensity not through volume or speed, but through intention and connection to your partner.

Some of us are more orally fixated than others. I wholeheartedly admit that I have an oral fixation. Many times I prefer giving a blow job or cunnilingus to penetrative sex. Here are a few general tips on the giving and receiving of oral stimulation.

Use your whole mouth—Explore your partner's body with your tongue, your lips, the back of your throat, the inside of your cheeks, and the wetness of your saliva.

Incorporate your whole body—Try fellating while looking up at your partner versus blindfolded. How is it different? How are your legs, toes, fingers, and arms engaged and connecting with your partner during the blow job? Try to bring a feeling of erotic energy from the tips of your toes to the crown of your head as your mouth meets your partner's cock or cunt. If you are receiving, try to feel your whole body alive and opening up as you actively receive sensation from your partner.

You are not a passive object or orifice—Let's toss out the stale idea that blow jobs are about being done or that women are holes to stick something into. Neither partner in a sexual scenario is passive. Both are active and actively engaging in mutual satisfaction for one another. It's not just about pleasing the other partner. Think: How can I please my mouth, my lips, my throat with my partner's cock?

Oral sex is not limited to the genitals—Oh, the many things that we can fellate and explore with our mouths! Fingers are a great body part to start with. Letting your tongue and lips explore your partner's digits can be a great way to connect and build intimacy while building erotic energy through oral stimulation. Fellating hands, high heels, boots, feet, food (bananas, lollipops, popsicles), or sex toys are all possibilities. Think of the many ways you can explore your partner's body with your mouth. Oral sex is not limited to the genitals. Visualize your mouth exploring and giving loving intimacy to your partner as you roam the landscape of your partner's body, the navel, up and down your partner's legs, back, thighs, anus, the back of the neck, clavicle, behind the ears. From sweet kisses to lapping, biting, and devouring your partner, you can explore a full range of sensations with your mouth.

Cotton candy and diamonds—When I was around twenty-four, I received some of the best oral sex advice that I've ever heard. I was on the set of a porn film and about to give my co-star a blow job. The director looked at me and said "I want to see you suck that cock like it's cotton candy and diamonds!" Not only does this sound hilarious, it made all the difference in my oral sex technique. I needed to shift my intent away from giving pleasure with my mouth. I was not only giving, but also receiving something sweet, delicious, rich, and luxurious. Before giving your next blow job, try visualizing yourself consuming the most delicious thing that you have ever put in your mouth. Something that is so delicious that you never want it to end. With every lap, you grow more and more ravenous for your partner. You want to lap and suck and caress every inch of your partner!

Giving Blow Jobs

Whether you are giving a blow job to a fleshy cock or a strap-on, these tips and techniques can add a variety of different pleasurable sensations to your sexy mama repertoire.

Keep your lips soft and pillowy. It's easy to tense your lips by wrapping them tightly around your teeth to prevent your teeth from scraping your partner's cock during a blow job, but this can be a less pleasurable sensation than keeping your lips soft. Practice with your fingers. Keep your lips loose, soft, wet, and round as they make their way up and down the head and shaft of your partner's cock.

Now, try extending your tongue and keeping your top lip soft and pillowy so that you are giving your partner the sensation of a luscious lip on top and a wet tongue on the bottom. I usually extend my thumb and support my tongue with it as I bob up and down on my partner's cock. This is a simple and effective technique that always gets a "Wow!" from my partners.

Try swirling your tongue around the head and shaft as you bob up and down. Vary your speed. There is no rush. Try not to get stuck in your head as you try these new techniques. Practicing on a sex toy or banana or even your fingers is a great way to develop muscle memory so that when you are alone with your partner you can be more relaxed.

On the underside of the head of the cock you will find a little V (if your partner is circumcised), or you will be able to see where the foreskin connects to the underside of the shaft near the tip (if your partner is uncircumcised). This little spot is very sensitive and has a lot of delicious nerve endings, and it can be an excellent spot to get to know. This area is called the *frenulum*. Try tonguing the frenulum while you look up and into your partner's eyes. You can try little circles or a broad flat tongue moving back and forth. You don't want to stay just in this one spot. In fact, with any of these tips and techniques, know that they are like different spices or different notes. You don't want to play just one single note or use one spice in a dish. Find the combination that works for you and your partner, or throw one of these techniques into your regular blow job and see how it amps things up. I often like to stimulate the frenulum and head of the cock, making eye contact, and then dip down, swallowing the entire cock.

It can also be really enjoyable to swirl your tongue around the entire head of the cock. The area where the head of the cock and shaft meet is sensitive as well. This area is called the *coronal ridge*. Using your hands, tongue, or lips to wrap around this spot can be a delicious experience. Try adding a little suction and pop your mouth off of the head, applying a little pressure around the coronal ridge. I like to call this the lollipop!

Many moms I meet want to explore deep-throating as a new oral sex technique. Deep-throating a cock can be fun, and it can be a new technique to add to your repertoire. But again, it's not the only technique you want to engage in. Add some variety.

If you would like to try deep-throating, practice first with a dildo or banana. I highly recommend the Vixen VixSkin dildo for deep throating. It's perfect because it has a cushy head, which is more comfortable for the throat. Start with a small dildo. If you need to work up toward a size that is closer to the size of your partner's cock, you can always get multiple dildos to practice on.

First, try to relax your throat. When we gag, it's because our throat muscles contract and tense up. We want to avoid tension. Tension is the enemy of sexual pleasure. Let tension go. Try some big full body yawns. Bring a mindfulness to how open and big and relaxed your throat muscles are right now. You want to experience that same openness when swallowing your partner's cock.

Insert the dildo into your mouth and find where your gag reflex kicks in. When you feel yourself start to gag or feel your throat muscles contract, back the dildo up a little. Now allow it to just hang out there. Relax your mouth around the cock and start to become comfortable with its presence. If you feel tension in your neck or shoulders, do some neck circles or shoulder rolls. Shake your tension out and release it. You are an empowered, sexy mama capable of gifting epic proportions of pleasure. You are engulfing your partner and swallowing your partner whole with your radical ecstasy. Slowly inch the dildo back farther, always backing up just a touch if you are gagging. By doing this you are training your throat muscles.

Experiment with positions. I enjoy either being on top of my partner or kneeling while my partner is standing if I'm going to be deep-throating. Retain some control of the situation and set boundaries. If you don't want your partner to hold your head while you are pleasuring your partner's cock, you can state that as a boundary. It's important that you feel comfortable, relaxed, and in control. Remember, you don't have to stay down long on the cock. I like to go all the way down to the base of the cock and then back up, allowing the shaft and head to pass through my lips.

Drool and saliva are okay! Wet sex is yummy! Drool and saliva help to lubricate the throat and allow the cock to slide down smoothly. In fact, I often like to deep throat pretty early in the blow job to develop some nice, viscous lubricant for the blow job. Keep hydrated so that you continue to produce saliva. And don't forget to breathe. Breath is a huge part of sex, regardless of the activity. You can breathe through your nose, through your mouth around your partner's cock, or while bobbing up and down. Another great time to breathe is when you take a moment to smile and look at your partner while you are stroking your partner's wet cock.

And what about receiving oral stimulation? How do we relax into oral sex and guide our partners through the way that we wish to be devoured? This is one of the concerns that I hear the most regarding oral sex—that individuals are so stumped about how to communicate with their partner about the way they want to be stimulated, and find such frustration in receiving stimulation that isn't arousing to them, that they would rather just bypass oral sex altogether. How do we receive with gratitude and guide our partners as we receive connection and intimacy with joy and pleasure?

Looking for ways to guide your partner toward more enjoyable oral sex? Here are some of my favorite techniques that I like to suggest to my partners when I'm receiving.

The most important thing is to keep it wet and passionate, and keep your mouth moving. If you are bored and just going through the motions, those emotional elements come across energetically in your sexual activities, and it can feel really disconnected.

Try lapping! That's right: Lap at your partner's vulva from bottom to top. You can try small laps and large, broad laps of the tongue. You can lap one side of the vulva and then the other, alternating tongue laps. You can even try broad tongue laps on and around the clitoris.

Keep moving. You can move your loose, wet lips and tongue around in circles or figure eights and even tease the clitoris or different areas of the vulva with your tongue. Try engulfing the vulva with your mouth and adding a little suction, or try penetrating the vagina with your tongue! Think of this as a grand exploration of your partner's cunt. Listen to your partner's body language. Is she pulling you near, or is her body not very reactive?

If you dive into cunnilingus right away, your partner might not experience the fireworks she was hoping for. Part of this is due to the fact that her vulva hasn't had time to warm up and become stimulated and engorged yet. Manual stimulation and vulval massage is a great way to bring blood to the genitals and increase engorgement and sensitivity. There is no rush. Take your time. Make out, watch porn, and start to explore one another's bodies. Maybe starting by stimulating her nipples with your mouth will give her body a chance to start to relax into an aroused state for more pleasurable cunnilingus.

CHAPTER

21

Kink

WHETHER YOU ARE PREGNANT, postpartum, or fully immersed
in motherhood, you might find yourself interested in exploring new and
adventurous elements of your sexual self. Our desires and sexual selves are
forever morphing and changing, and during the transitions of pregnancy
and motherhood, we can sometimes find that these desires and cravings
surprise us or lead us outside of our familiar palette of sexual practices.
Even if you have been a longtime sexual adventurer and edge player, you
might find yourself consistently redefining your boundaries and accessing
your desires during this transformative time in your life.

Personally, I have always enjoyed a lot of sensation, tight bondage, and
hard impact play, but as I approached the end of my second trimester, I
discovered that my body was really craving a sensual touch. Massage and
light touch actually felt really good, when typically I found those types
of touch to be annoying. I was dreadfully worried at the time that this
was a permanent transition into "weakness." I was wrong. My body and
my desire were just shifting around. I was getting a chance to explore
the softer side of Madison Young. It was an interesting and challenging
practice in following the ebb and flow and needs of my body and desire.
Nothing is static, and certainly not our identities. Honestly, I believe that
so many of my resources were going to making my little bambino that

I needed to be nurtured more than I needed to explore the edges of my endurance in a sexual capacity.

In this chapter you will find an introduction to a few of the adventurous elements of sexual desire that you might find yourself interested in exploring during your journey into motherhood.

Kink and BDSM can be a fun and exciting way to explore new sensations and new sexual connections with your partner in brand-new ways. If you are a mom looking to explore kink in your love life, I highly recommend seeking out your local BDSM community. Attending BDSM workshops with your loved one can be an exciting way to take on a new sexual adventure together and gather the skills and experience you need to venture forward safely. There are also excellent online resources, such as kinkuniversity.com and kinkacademy.com. A simple yet effective tool for starting an exploration of kink is a blindfold. Simply taking away sight can present a new level of vulnerability and will amp up the intensity of even the smallest touch.

If you are currently pregnant and interested in kink, whether you are a seasoned practitioner or trying it out for the first time, make sure to use your best judgment and consult your doctor before engaging in any potentially risky activity. Remember, there is a lot going on with your body during pregnancy. You are building another human! And that can throw off your balance, totally change your blood circulation, and disorient you, among other things. These don't always pair well with certain kink and bondage activities that require balance or that restrict blood circulation. That said, as a longtime bondage enthusiast, I engaged in modified bondage and kink activities throughout my pregnancy.

International BDSM educator, performer, and ER nurse Shay Tiziano shares with us her experience and expertise on navigating pregnancy and a kinky sex life. You can find more about Shay at her Web site, www.stefanosandshay.com.

PREGNANCY AND BDSM
WITH SHAY TIZIANO

The idea of a pregnant woman being tied up and flogged is almost certain to evoke complicated emotions and concerns from observers, dungeon monitors (DMs), and of course the players themselves! It's easy to say (or imply) that women should just stop playing during their pregnancies, but that approach lacks nuance and a consideration of the realities of kinky play and healthy pregnancy. This section is intended to offer some information on playing as safely as possible during a healthy pregnancy, and is intended both for the players and for the information of DMs and spectators. Most of this section addresses bottoming during pregnancy, simply because that is where I've heard people express the most concern about safety.

Note that any sort of high-risk pregnancy (pre-eclampsia, incompetent cervix, gestational diabetes, etc.) is beyond the scope of this text; please ask your doctor about specific activity limitations in those cases.

Pain and Sensation Play

In a healthy pregnancy, there shouldn't be issues with most sensation play (light to moderate flogging on the upper back and buttocks, wax play, etc.). Many women find that their skin is more sensitive during pregnancy, so a pregnant bottom may find that she doesn't have the pain tolerance she once did. Of course, stay away from any kind of impact on the belly—not a major part of most people's BDSM repertoires anyway and therefore probably fairly easy to avoid. A pregnant woman's body is designed to protect the developing baby; generally, an injury has to be severe enough to seriously injure the woman before the fetus is harmed. The walls of the uterus are thick, strong muscle, and the baby is floating in a cushion of amniotic fluid. While miscarriage is quite common, especially in early pregnancy, trauma is a very rare cause of fetal demise. Chromosomal abnormalities, smoking, drugs, and maternal health issues such as diabetes are much more frequent causes of miscarriage. However, during the third trimester, a direct blow to the abdomen can cause the placenta to separate from the uterus, causing a life-threatening emergency for both the mother and the baby. Consider the abdomen a no-go area for any sort of impact play for the duration of the pregnancy.

Good places for mild to moderate impact play during pregnancy include the back, butt, and thighs. Keep in mind that pregnancy involves frequent visits to the OB-GYN. While I encourage you to be "out" to your doctor, I think even the most open-minded MD is at the least going to give you major side-eye if you come in for a prenatal check with huge bruises and abrasions. Additionally, pregnant women are more likely to scar, so that's a consideration anytime you may break skin. Use common sense in your play.

Of course, there are the boobs—oh, how the boobs change during the pregnancy/birth/breastfeeding process! Often one of the first symptoms of pregnancy is extreme sensitivity in the nipples. So you may find yourself retiring the clover clamps for the duration of the pregnancy—and probably far longer, if you will be breastfeeding. Somewhere in the third trimester, the milk factory starts cooking. Breasts start secreting colostrum, or pre-milk, a clear, yellowish sweet-tasting liquid. Around that time, I started warning my partners "Hey, those work" when they would go to suck on my breasts. Best to advise people that they are about to encounter bodily fluids they may not have expected! Everyone's experience varies. Just speaking for myself, even many years after my last pregnancy I'm no longer into nipple or breast play. It's not that my breasts "belong to baby" or anything like that. While I was breastfeeding (for a total of more than three years), my boobs were getting messed with for at least two hours a day. I find that I'm "full up" on any sort of boob stimulation. Maybe they'll eventually become an erogenous zone again, but I'm not counting on it.

Blood and Blood Clots

Blood volume increases during pregnancy. While the number of red blood cells (responsible for carrying nutrients and oxygen) goes up during pregnancy, the volume of plasma (the liquid component of blood) goes up even more. Because of this, pregnant women have a functional type of anemia (low blood count). Furthermore, hormonal changes tend to lead to decreases in average blood pressure, with the lowest blood pressure usually occurring around twenty-eight weeks. Pregnant women are therefore at increased risk of significant blood pressure drops, which may lead to dizziness and fainting. BDSM play (topping or bottoming) may exacerbate this, especially if combined with dehydration.

The changes in blood volume and flow may also affect a woman's comfort in certain positions. In the later stages of pregnancy, the uterus may put pressure on the inferior vena cava (the large vein that carries blood back to the heart from the legs). In the supine position (lying on the

back), this decrease in blood return can become significant, leading to greater risk of dizziness or discomfort
during prolonged periods of lying on the back.

Pregnant women are prone to blood clots, and
prolonged periods of immobility can cause blood to pool
and make clots more likely to form. Therefore, while light
bondage with some "wiggle room" is perfectly okay during
pregnancy, extreme or immobilizing bondage should be
avoided.

Bondage

The American Congress of Obstetricians and Gynecologists recommends that pregnant women avoid activities
that put them "at high risk of falling" (including downhill
skiing and horseback riding). The question of what bondage
activities constitute "high fall risk" is perhaps so subjec-
tive as to be useless in this discussion. However, there
are a number of more specific concerns with bondage
during pregnancy, particularly when it comes to suspension. As mentioned above, tight and immobilizing bondage
should be avoided due to risk of blood clots. Bondage that
restricts the chest or breathing (as suspension often does)
would be a particular concern. (See the following section
on breathing issues for details.) Hormonal changes during
pregnancy cause the ligaments and joints to become more
relaxed and mobile, and they can be more prone to injury.
The body's center of balance is changed, which can cause
balance problems and back pain. Pregnant women are
often advised to avoid full inversion. Face-up suspension
would be concerning due to pressure on the vena cava.
My overall assessment is that I would certainly not tell a
pregnant woman she can't be suspended, but she needs

a lot of body awareness and a skilled rigger who is knowl-
edgeable about the physiological changes of pregnancy.

Breathing Issues

There are a multitude of changes that occur to the
upper respiratory tract during pregnancy, all designed to
improve oxygen flow to meet the needs of both mother
and fetus. Pregnant women have a decreased ability to
adapt to low oxygen levels and therefore will become
distressed much more rapidly during breath play. Because
of potential risks to both mother and fetus, I recommend
avoiding breath play altogether during pregnancy.

Fainting and near-fainting are not uncommon during
pregnancy. If you are feeling faint or dizzy, lie down on
your left side. If a pregnant woman has fainted, immediately lay her down on her left side in the recovery position
(unless there is concern about trauma, in which case, call
911).

Electrical/Fire Play

There isn't a whole lot of data on electrical safety in
pregnancy. In the medical literature relating to pregnant
women, electrical injuries typically produce damage due
to burns, electrical damage to the heart, or muscle injuries due to the spasms that go along with exposure to
electrical currents. The standard advisories for playing
safely with electricity (avoid application to the face or
across the heart) apply to pregnant women. Additionally,
the amniotic fluid in which the fetus lies conducts electricity well. Because the fetus is essentially surrounded
by a conducting medium, I recommend avoiding pelvic
or abdominal application of electricity during pregnancy.

Using a violet wand or TENS unit on the extremities is still fine.

Burns can be very serious injuries in pregnant women, although typically a large surface area needs to be affected before major consequences to the fetus occur. The general safety rules (short duration of exposure, accessibility of fire blankets, etc.) should be followed while pregnant.

Penetration during Pregnancy

Vaginal and anal penetration during pregnancy are generally safe up until the water breaks. (If there is any doubt, ask your doctor!) I bottomed in a fisting scene when I was eight months pregnant. I did quite a bit of research first, including asking my labor and delivery nurse friend for advice, and the consensus was that as long as my cervix was still closed and my water was not broken, fisting was no problem at all. As a side note, I didn't require any sutures after my delivery (didn't tear at all!), so maybe fisting is a good pre-game warm-up, as it were? It's a bit similar to the perineal massage that obstetricians recommend.

Public Scenes

If you'll be playing in a public dungeon, keep in mind that seeing a pregnant woman in a scene does tend to throw the dungeon monitors for a loop—many of them are completely flummoxed. So, if you're going to do a public scene while pregnant, I'd recommend checking in with the DM and/or host first (always a good idea anyway), describing the scene and explaining that it's safe for you to do it. That way you can avoid scaring people and potentially having your scene interrupted by a concerned DM.

Topping while Pregnant

For the pregnant top, the first adjustment you may have to make is to your wardrobe. Due to changes in the back and hips during pregnancy, high heels are not recommended. Of course, this applies to bottoms as well—those stilettos will have to go into storage for a bit! Additionally, many women find they tire very easily during pregnancy, especially in the first and third trimesters. So you may want to plan scenes somewhat less ambitious than your usual triathlon of pain. This would be a very good time for pregnant tops to break out the lazy dom toys—things like TENS or other electrical units, needles, urethral sounds, clothespins, rubber bands—anything you can use while standing still, or even sitting down! Women generally feel clumsy and less coordinated in the later stages of pregnancy, and the incidence of injury (falls, twisted ankles, etc.) increases. Keep this in mind when planning your play.

Psychological Considerations

Emotionally, pregnancy can be dangerous terrain. The potent hormone cocktail necessary to maintain the pregnancy and support the growing fetus can cause moodiness, crying spells, feelings of protectiveness (both of the baby and one's mate), anxiety, and vulnerability. While humiliation play may have previously been very erotic, a pregnant woman may find that it now just reduces her to tears, and not in a good way. Of course this is going to be very individual, and something that will require constant communication and ongoing negotiation. For myself, I got more toppy throughout my pregnancy. My partner, Stefanos, called it "going into mama lion mode."

Conclusions

Keep standard warning signs in mind. If you have vaginal bleeding or haven't felt any fetal movement, see a doctor. If this is your first pregnancy, enjoy the ability to go out and play without having to worry about all the logistics (babysitter, having enough milk in the fridge, etc.) that have to be dealt with after the baby's born! Your life won't be over—it will just be more complicated and much busier.

Open Relationships

Open relationships are a common topic among parents who attend my workshops and who I work with in my coaching practice. Many people—no matter where they might be in their relationship—find the idea of having more than one sexual partner exciting, or find that it's something that they would like to try out. For some people this might look like more of a one-time sexual experience; for others it might mean going to sex parties where you engage in sexual play with others; for still others it might mean having more than one partner. Sexy mamas and sexuality and wellness experts Eri Kardos and Cara Kelsey share with us their experiences in practicing open relationships during pregnancy and motherhood and the challenges and successes that they encountered during their experience.

Eri: Being pregnant definitely made an impact on how I navigated poly dynamics within my relationships. I found that I needed far more "me" time than in the past. I also needed to be nurtured and have my body cared for while I grew this little life inside of me. This meant that more of my free time went towards journaling or getting a massage instead of going out on a date with a significant other. Basically, I needed to take myself on more dates! When I did have time with partners, I experienced a shift from my more masculine energy (driving forward, initiating activities, etc.) to a more feminine energy (holding space, exploring creativity, etc.). For the first time in my life, I didn't enjoy driving a car. I wanted my partners to take me places, plan quiet evenings together, and sweetly love on my body. Life began to slow down a bit, and I first experienced it internally before it leaked out into my partnerships and then impacted the rest of my life. Prior to being pregnant, I had many play partners in addition to my main squeezes. These partnerships slowly came to an end, and I chose not to pursue others. I turned my focus inward toward myself and my family.

These changes opened opportunities for depth and playing with energy in a new way within our family. It was difficult at first, yet slowly became easier with time. I believe that pregnancy and labor are a sacred rite of passage for women. You will never be the same after it. This can be startling for your relationships and can impact your open structure in big, unforeseen ways.

Now that I am a mom, I have a new primary partner. He is a whopping ten and a half pounds and I am madly in love with him. It has been more challenging to balance all the other aspects of life, and I love figuring it out anew each week. I am experiencing a disconnect from my two main partners, especially in the sexual realm. It is incredibly important to set time aside for a weekly date and have someone watch your child. At first I thought we could simply have sex when the baby was asleep. Nope! Every time he stirs or makes any sound whatsoever, my mom brain is focused on him (see: not sexy).

In addition, time is different. I move on his schedule. The best time for a date is in the afternoon or just after dinner when he is napping. No more late nights for me, so we need to be creative about when we see our partners.

One other really important aspect to consider is how to prepare metamours (that is, your partner's partners) for the arrival of the baby. My metamour happens to live in our house with us. Prior to baby, she and my husband spent four nights a week together. Post-baby, I needed daddy upstairs helping me through the long nights for the first three months. This really put a strain on their relationship. I am so grateful to have her help with the house and caring for the baby. I cannot imagine trying to be a mom with less than six adults chipping in! Yay, poly!

I fell in love with my other life partner (my husband being my first) while pregnant. On our first date I was already three months pregnant. I had thought that being pregnant would scare potential lovers and part-ners off, but I think it simply attracted a new breed of person. The ones I connected deeply with during pregnancy were risk-takers and had an interest in having children. I was filled to the brim with creative energy, and starting a new, intense relationship seemed perfectly fitting while pregnant.

If you are interested in exploring an open relationship for the first time during pregnancy, I encourage you to check in with your heart. Do you have space for another love in your life? Will they have the emotional maturity to support you through this time and also give you space once your baby arrives? Will you have enough time and energy to grow with your current partner and help your partner move into a parenting space?

A few other tips: First, educate yourself about STI transmission and make choices that will not add worry to your pregnancy. I was far less slutty during pregnancy to avoid exposing my child to unnecessary risk. There are still so many wonderful ways to explore your sexy side while pregnant without a lot of health risks.

Second, open relationships require incredible communication skills. Make sure you and your beloveds are all on the same page and learning new skills on a regular basis. A third-party professional coach or therapist is encouraged.

Third, choose people who genuinely love children. It is one thing to care for your own child; it is another to care for someone else's child.

Fourth, pregnant sex is fun! It requires a bit more creativity, especially in the third trimester, and it is so worth it. Be prepared for new discov-eries about your body every week, and be gentle with yourself as you take on this momentous project.

Finally, don't fool yourself into thinking this is going to be as simple and easy as *Full House* makes it look. Adding more people to your family is challenging. If you are looking to explore an open relationship while pregnant or as a mom, you are really adding to the complexity. This will not solve any issues you have in your current relationship. Be ready to dig in deep and learn a whole lot about yourself and how to communicate your wants and needs.

As a mom, I am now loving having multiple partners and metamours. Everyone in our family is incredibly supportive of me and takes care of my baby. Our house mantra is "outnumber the children," and our little village is succeeding at raising a wonderful child in a loving environment.

I am an international communications coach, and my work focuses on helping people communicate more effectively, both personally and professionally. All that being said, the changes in hormones and lifestyle that come with pregnancy and motherhood really put my tools and skills to the test. Here are my tips:

First, I encourage people with intimate relationships to learn a new conflict resolution tool. Some that I recommend include Hendrix's Imago Dialogue, Rosenberg's Nonviolent Communication, or Gottman's Aftermath of a Fight or Regrettable Incident. This will help break old patterns of conflict resolution and really get to the heart of the matter together.

Second, pick out a hand signal or safe word for calling a timeout when emotions are escalating. I found that my emotions were just a bit heightened and unpredictable during pregnancy and immediately afterward. It was really helpful for all partners involved to have a clear way to pause a bubbling fight and get space before applying one of the tools mentioned above.

Third, I encourage people to read *Raising an Emotionally Intelligent Child* by John Gottman. It is a great tool for helping teach your children (and most adults!) healthy ways of connecting to and communicating their emotions and needs.

Fourth, check out Betty Martin's "Wheel of Consent" at www. bettymartin.org/videos. I had a hard time asking for what I needed and receiving care when I was pregnant. This model really helped me move into a place of grounded understanding and communication, even when it was tough to ask for help.

Finally, I encourage you to find a parenting support group. It will help normalize your experience and give you more space to ask for what you need. Plus, you'll learn all sorts of tribal knowledge about how to survive this new phase of life.

Cara: My partner and I were nonmonogamous in some way or another for about three years before I got pregnant. We went to a lot of kinky and poly parties and were pretty settled in our sexy way of living. Pregnancy definitely put a hold on that for us. I was very sick during my whole first trimester and into my second, and had migraines and sciatica during my second trimester. During my third trimester I was diagnosed with preeclampsia and was told to take it super easy. Even a long walk could cause me to get dizzy and start to pass out. My body grew and became unfamiliar. I had a super hard time feeling sexy at all during pregnancy. Sex was hard for me even with my primary partner, so sex with other people was out of the question. I was insecure and trying to figure out how to love my new self. Because I was so insecure and felt so vulnerable with all of my health concerns, I was not super comfortable with my partner having other partners or exploring others sexually. He understood that and was very patient with me as we tried to figure out a new sexual rhythm for our relationship. I would also buy him erotic or sensual massages whenever we had extra money. I am a firm believer in sex work and the need for it, and this seemed like a great option for us. Paying for sex meant that when I was not feeling sexy at all, my partner could be fulfilled, and because it was a business transaction, I had no worries about a relationship forming. It gave us time to work together and gave me time to work with myself on a new and more complex sexual relationship.

After having my little one, it took a while to get back into nonmonogamy. I didn't feel like I had the emotional energy for other relationships. For months afterward, I rarely felt like being touched, but my sexuality was important to me. Now that I was healthy and able again, I needed to reclaim my body and my new sexual identity. My partner and I started having sex as soon as my doctor gave us the okay. We would have a close friend babysit for a couple hours and get a hotel or go to private hot tubs instead of doing dinner. This allowed me to get dressed up and go out knowing that my little one would be taken care of. As I got more comfortable touching myself and having sex with my partner regularly again, sex parties became more of an option. The more comfortable I became at sex parties, the more the idea of multiple partners became exciting again. My little one is three now, and my partner and I have spent a lot of time figuring out and negotiating what works for all of us in our nonmonogamous relationship. Dating takes a lot of energy, and we have to be realistic about how much of that energy we want to give to other people. Full disclosure with the people we date (and each other) is a must. Before a first date, I let my date know that I have a primary partner and a toddler. We both mostly date casually now, and sometimes we date other couples so that we are connecting with each other as well as other people. We negotiate for time a lot. There have been times when my partner has a lot of dates lined up and I don't, or the other way around, and we have to talk about that to make sure everyone feels taken care of. We have had to allow for a lot of fluidity in the spectrum of nonmonogamy. Sometimes I am just seeing women, sometimes we are fully open, and at other times we do group sex and sex with others only at parties. It depends on what is going on in our lives and how we are doing and feeling. My partner and I have full lives, so we don't date all the time. Sometimes I meet someone and I can't see him or her for a month because I am accommodating my job, my partner's job, friends, events that we have planned with our daughter, and many other things. Babysitters are expensive, but it is important for us. We try to go out together at least twice a month, and as a family once a week. From there, we can fill in time for individual dates and other events or priorities.

I would define and specify what you want out of an open relationship and go from there. Do you want to have casual sex with other people, group sex, relationships? What does that look like to you? The more specific and honest you are, the better. Start simple—maybe find a local sex party or look on a dating website. Jealousy does happen, so be prepared to own it, deal with it, and communicate about your feelings. If you are interested in threesomes or group sex, consider hiring an escort or professional. Look online for local workshops or discussion groups about different types of open relationships. Not only will you learn something, but it is a good way to meet other people. Be prepared to negotiate. Think about time—time for self-care, for your primary partner, and for your little one—and go from there. Think about energy: Do you have it? What do you need and want, what does your partner need and want, and what, in reality, can you achieve right now? Don't get attached to labels, and allow for fluidity—everything is allowed on the table for negotiation as long as you're willing to hear "no." There is always time for renegotiating!

Nonmonogamy can be very exciting and can allow for more open, honest communication and trust in a relationship. It can bring out your best and the best in your relationship, and it can bring out the worst—but as with anything, the more work you are willing to do on yourself and your relationship, the greater the reward!

It has become vital to be straightforward and specific in my communication. I cannot waste time or emotional energy on games or trying to read someone's mind. It took me a long time in my life to find my "no" and to listen to and voice my needs. As a mom, I have learned to be more assertive. I have become a much better communicator and much less concerned with whether people like me or not. Meditation has always been important to me, and I make sure that I am continuing to meditate as well as taking inventory of my day. Was I the person I want to be today? How can I do better tomorrow? Taking breaths when I am angry or nervous is something I am constantly doing and trying to teach my daughter to do. Writing down what I want or what I need has always been helpful with separating the chatter in my head from what is really important. A lot of times I will ask my partner for space during an argument or talk so I can sit with what I am feeling and figure out what I need. I spend a majority of my time trying to nurture and raise a tiny human, so making sure that my cup is full has to be a priority. If I am not taking time out of the day or week to work out or do something creative or loving for myself, I am doing myself and my daughter a huge injustice. Asking for what I want and asking for help has become easier because it is vital.

References

Muench MV and Canterino JC. "Trauma in pregnancy." *Obstetrics and Gynecology Clinics of North America* 2007; 34:555-83.

The American Congress of Obstetricians & Gynecologists, http://m.acog.org/

Stone, C. Keith, and Roger L. Humphries, eds. 2011. *CURRENT Diagnosis & Treatment Emergency Medicine*, 7th ed. New York: McGraw-Hill.

Afterword

LET'S ALL TAKE A big exhale. We just experienced quite a journey together, and I'm so grateful that I had the opportunity to be there beside you during this very special and intimate time in your life. As a writer and educator, I feel so full of gratitude that I am able to hold space and share my intimate experiences and journey with my community, and that I'm given the opportunity to hold space for others to share, communicate, and process their emotional experiences, transformative experiences, and intimate adventures and challenges.

Know that in this life, in this journey, we are all united, tethered, and connected through our shared experiences and celebrated in our expression of differences. Know that you are not alone, and that you deserve pleasure, and that loving ourselves serves as the foundation for modeling and guiding our children through a lifelong journey of pursuing their own passions and expressing love and connection with the friends and lovers that will one day come into their life.

This morning, my child asked me, "Mom, do you always have to be beautiful?" I responded with, "I do like to feel beautiful. Feeling beautiful for me means doing things that make me feel happy or wearing colors that make me smile or that make me feel confident or cozy when I'm wearing or surrounded by them. Being me."

Every day, find your beauty. Seek out what makes you happy. Do you need a wellness advocate? Recruit a friend, visit a mom's group, find a therapist that you like. Having an advocate can help us see through the haze and find small ways to add beauty, connection, and pleasure back to our lives.

We can be beautiful in all states of existence—without sleep, with kid snot on our sweater, and when we are changing diapers. Find the beauty in life, surrender to the moment, and seek the care and connection you need to fill your vessel with the love and beauty you deserve.

We are all forever changing, transforming, and evolving, and there is an absolute beauty in this.

Resources

Parenting Coaches, Therapists, and Sex Educators

Eri Kardos (www.erikardos.com)—Relationship and communication coach as well as sex educator.

Jamye Waxman (jamyewaxman.com)—Sex educator, mama, and author.

Kink Aware Professionals (ncsfreedom.org)—An amazing resource for finding physicians, psychologists, therapists, life coaches, and health and wellness practitioners who are "kink aware" and versed in alternative sexuality communities and lifestyles.

Natashia Fuksman (www.natashiafuksman.com)—Natashia is a psychotherapist working in the Bay Area. Her site has myriad resources listed for new mothers as well as workshops and new mom's groups that she facilitates.

San Francisco Sex Information Hotline (sfsi.org)—This is a national sex information hotline run by SFSI-trained sex educators. You can email them sex-related questions at ask-us@sfsi.org or call at 415-989-SFSI.

Savvy Parenting (www.savvyparentingsupport.com)—With offerings like online courses in early potty learning and sleep-savvy coaching, as well as individualized coaching sessions and consultations—and blog posts—Savvy Parenting is a wealth of knowledge and resources for parents.

Blogs and Magazines

Hip Mama (www.hipmamazine.com)—The original alternative parenting magazine.

How Great Sex Made Me a Good Mom (howgreatsexmademeagoodmom.com)—Shar Rednour's humorous, candid, and personal essays and advice can be found at this smart and witty blog.

Mutha Magazine (muthamagazine.com)—A brilliant online magazine for modern radical mamas, founded by Michelle Tea.

Rad Dad (www.raddadzine.blogspot.com)—A totally rad zine (and book) produced by writer, community organizer, and rad dad Tomas Moniz.

Sex Positive Parenting (thesexpositiveparent.com)—An excellent blog on sex-positive parenting by Airial Clark, MA, offering articles, classes, workshops, coaching, counseling, and consulting.

Susie Bright (susiebright.blogs.com)—Brilliant sex writer. Check out her mother/daughter sex advice, written with her daughter, Aretha Bright.

Maternity and Nursing Lingerie

Bella Materna—www.bellamaterna.com

Cake Maternity—www.cakematernity.com

Destination Maternity—www.destinationmaternity.com (Dita Von Teese's nursing bra, Von Follies, is available at this website)

Fig Leaves—www.figleaves.com

Hot Milk—www.hotmilklingerie.com

You Lingerie—www.you-lingerie.com

Talking with Kids about Sex, Gender Expression, Bodies, and Reproduction

Books

10,000 Dresses by Marcus Ewert and Rex Ray

Morris Micklewhite and the Tangerine Dress by Christine Baldacchino

My Princess Boy by Cheryl Kilodavis (myprincessboy.com)

Once Upon a Potty by Alona Frankel

Sex is a Funny Word: A Book about Bodies, Feelings, and You by Cory Silverberg

What Makes a Baby by Cory Silverberg

Websites

Gender Spectrum—www.genderspectrum.org

Our Family Coalition—www.ourfamily.org

Scarleteen—www.scarleteen.com

Sex Education

Looking for hot and sexy sex education videos to watch with your partner to inspire some heat in the bedroom? Check out these websites:

Kink Academy—kinkacademy.com

Kink University—kinkuniversity.com

Passionate U—passionateu.com

Pleasure Ed—goodvibrationsvod.com

Vivid Ed—vivid-ed.com

Sex-Positive Sex Toy Stores

Babeland—babeland.com

Early to Bed—early2bed.com

Good for Her—goodforher.com

Good Vibrations—goodvibes.com

Pleasure Chest—thepleasurechest.com

SheBop—shebptheshop.com

BreastFeeding Support and Education

La Leche League—lalecheleague.org

LLL Breastfeeding Helpline—breastfeedinghelpline.com

Loving Support Breastfeeding Program—lovingsupport.org

Contributor Bios

ANYA DE MONTIGNY is a sex educator, coach, and master body-worker with over eighteen years of experience working with individuals, couples, and groups. Anya has credentials as a sex educator, clinical sexologist, certified sexological bodyworker, bondassage trainer, tantra yoga teacher, and certified massage therapist. Anya combines her classroom training with her years of hands on work to bring to the public the best in adult sex education..

ASHLEY PIA grew up in Marin County, California, and has been a makeup artist for thirteen years. Now, at the age of thirty-two, she is raising a seventeen-month-old daughter with her partner of ten years. They love camping, making jewelry, and DIY projects. Ashley is currently obsessed with her daughter Chloe.

AYA DE LEON is a writer and performer working in poetry, fiction, and hip hop theater. Her work has received acclaim in the *Village Voice,* the *Washington Post,* and *American Theatre Magazine* and has been featured on Def Poetry, in *Essence* magazine, and in various anthologies and journals. She was named Best Discovery in Theater by the *San Francisco Chronicle* in 2004 for *Thieves in the Temple: The Reclaiming of Hip Hop,* a solo show about fighting sexism and commercialism in hip hop. Also in 2004, she received a Goldie award in spoken word from the *San Francisco Bay Guardian* for *Thieves* and her subsequent show *Aya de Leon Is Running for President.* In 2005 she was voted Slamminest Poet in the *East Bay Express.* Aya has been an artist-in-residence at Stanford University, a Cave Canem poetry fellow, and a slam poetry champion. She publicly married herself in the nineties and since 1995 has been hosting an annual Valentine's Day show that focuses on selflove. She has released three spoken word CDs, several chapbooks, and a video of *Thieves*. Since becoming a mom in 2009, she has been transitioning from being a touring performer into being a novelist. Aya is the director of the Poetry for the People program founded by June Jordan at the University of California, Berkeley, teaching poetry, spoken word, and hip hop.

CARA KELSEY is a certified massage therapist as well as a certified sexual health educator. She is a mother, a partner, a pleasure enthusiast, and an overall sex nerd. She is currently doing Mama Massages with two organizations in Berkeley, California, and has been involved with many sex related workshops and classes in San Francisco.

CARLIN ROSS is an attorney, entrepreneur, and keeper of all things Betty Dodson. She's the editor-in-chief of their website (dodsonandross. com), co-leader of their Bodysex workshops and certification program, and the president of the Betty A. Dodson Foundation. She hails from Brooklyn and is happiest at the park with her son, Grayson, and her husband, Steve.

CARLYLE JANSEN is the founder of Good for Her, Toronto's premier sexuality shop and workshop center (which sometimes feels like her firstborn child). She is also the producer of the Feminist Porn Awards. She has two boys whom she had on her own before meeting her life partner. Carlyle has been teaching workshops and coaching individuals and couples since 1995 and is a guest speaker at the Guelph Sex Therapy Intensive Training and many university programs. She writes a column in both *Tonic* and *Her* magazine and is interviewed regularly by media and documentaries. She has authored two books: *Sex Yourself: The Woman's Guide to Mastering Masturbation and Achieving Powerful Orgasms* and *Anal Sex Basics: The Beginner's Guide to Maximizing Anal Pleasure for Every Body*. She also wrote the chapter on Sensational Oral Sex in *Secrets of the Sex Masters*. She loves helping others have (even) better sex!

CAROLINE RHAME graduated from Mount Holyoke College with a degree in art history after taking a year abroad in Florence, Italy, studying at the Lorenzo de' Medici School. She worked at magazines in New York City, including *Cosmopolitan* and *Marie Claire*. She is now a writer of historical erotica and lives in the San Francisco East Bay with her two daughters and husband.

ERI KARDOS is an international communications coach, speaker, wife, partner, and mom based in Seattle. She specializes in empowering people to choose their own adventure in relationships, career, and life. As an educator, she teaches personal selfdevelopment workshops and private coaching sessions on a wide variety of topics, including communication and consent through self-awareness, conflict resolution, ethical nonmonogamy, marriage preparation, and exploring intimacy. On the business side, she uses her MBA and background at a Fortune 100 company to teach professional skills including networking, interviewing, and performance management. A certified Integral Coach, Eri provides video coaching to clients across the globe. In September 2015 she became the mother of Aavi. Together they have traveled thousands of miles, connecting with their global community and exploring this big world. You can find her online at www.erikardos.com or follow her on LinkedIn, Twitter (@ Eri_Kardos), and Facebook (www.facebook.com/erikardoscoaching).

HARMONY NILES is the mother of a strong-willed three-year-old. She spent her pre-motherhood days selling wine and managing busy restaurants. Now she is pursuing a graduate degree in social work, with a dream of helping teenage girls develop a healthy relationship to their sexuality.

ISABELLE BOESCH is the mother of two beautiful, divine children (four-and-a-half-year-old Grace and three-month-old Ben) who rock her world and still have the ability to take her breath away. She is perceptive and intuitive, and she mothers with heart. She is an advocate for mothering arts with her MomME Circles (www.mommecircle.com) and has taught yoga to mothers and children for the past ten years. Some days she can be found dancing with her family, even though her rhythm has long ago left the building. Other days you will find her simply staring at her family in awe.

JARDANA PEACOCK is a holistic healer and embodied leadership coach who works with change makers intentionally. She recently released an ebook, *Heal Myself, Heal the World: Practices for Liberation,* where she chronicles her life, journey into social justice activism and healing, and lessons learned from over fifteen years of spiritual and wellness practice and work. Her writing has also been featured in the *Huffington Post, Decolonizing Yoga,* and the *Feminist Wire.* She is based in Nashville, Tennessee, where she lives with her partner and two sons. She can be reached at www.jardanapeacock.com.

JAMYE WAXMAN, M.ED., is a mother, sex educator, writer, and aspiring therapist. Jamye is also the author of the books *How to Break Up with Anyone: Letting Go of Friends, Family, and Everyone In-Between, Hot Sex: Over 200 Things You Can Try Tonight!* (coauthored with Emily Morse), and *Getting Off: A Woman's Guide to Masturbation.* Follow her on Twitter (@jamye) and Facebook (www.facebook.com/jamye-waxman).

LUCKY TOMASZEK is a sexuality educator living with her three kids in Milwaukee, Wisconsin. In addition to her current role as education coordinator at The Tool Shed, Cream City's only feminist sex toy store, she has a long background as a birth worker and parenting columnist. Most mornings you can find her balancing her cat and her keyboard in her lap while doggedly trying to make the world a smarter, safer place for people of all genders, orientations, and relationship groupings.

MOOREA MALATT is a parent educator, parent coach, and workshop and event speaker. She is the founder of www.savvyparentingsupport.com, a gentle and natural-minded online resource for early parenting challenges. Moorea is an expert in gentle (and early) potty learning, gentle sleep learning, and gentle discipline and the author of online learning programs, books, and articles. She leads soldout workshops and provides private phone consultations for naturally minded parents of kiddos from newborns to age four. She loves being on podcasts, speaking at summits, and giving talks at baby fairs.

NATASHIA FUKSMAN, MA, LMFT is a practicing therapist and group facilitator in the Bay Area. With over twenty years of experience working with individuals, couples, and families, Natashia's main focus has been on working with parents, with a keen focus on transitions in identity as they relate to our intimate relationships and cultural background. Originally from New York City, Natashia is the featured doula and childbirth educator in the documentary *The Business of Being Born.* She has served on the boards of DONA International, the Childbirth Education Association of Metropolitan New York, Postpartum Support International, and BirthWays. She is the founding director of the NYC Doula Collective and the former doula trainer for the New York Open Center. Aside from her private practice, Natashia is a founding co-director of Rockridge Wellness Center, a facilitator with Oakland Mom2Mom, and the head facilitator of Living Room: Women's Meditation and Conversation, an open weekly gathering for women to convene and share their experiences as mothers and beyond. Natashia offers talks and workshops relating to sexuality, cultural identity, and parenthood throughout the Bay Area. Natashia is the mother of two beautiful boys. She grew up trilingual, with family roots in Eastern Europe and Brazil.

SEARAH DEYSACH owns Chicago's feminist sex shop, Early to Bed, and loves sex education, reproductive justice, her kid, and her spouse.

SHAR REDNOUR coauthored (with Carol Queen, PhD) *The Sex & Pleasure Book: Good Vibrations Guide to Great Sex for Everyone* (www. thesexandpleasurebook.com); she wrote the parenting sections. In Jiz Lee's *Coming Out Like a Porn Star: Essays on Pornography, Protection, and Privacy* she writes candidly about how being the daughter of sex-positive, working-class parents affected her as a mom. She has two forthcoming parenting books, including *How Great Sex Made Me a Good Mom,* based on her blog of the same name. Her book *The Femme's Guide to the Universe* is available on www.audible.com. She was proud to be selected to narrate the audiobook version of the biography *Bad Girls Go Everywhere: The Life of Helen Gurley Brown* by Jennifer Scanlon. Details of her work at *On Our Backs*, Fatale Media, and S.I.R. Video Productions can be found in *New Views on Pornography: Sexuality, Politics, and the Law,* edited by Lynn Comella and Shira Tarrant. Shar cowrote and directed the educational DVD *Healing Sex: The Complete Guide to Sexual Wholeness* featuring Staci Haines.

SHAY TIZIANO is an ER nurse and international BDSM educator and performer. Shay and her partner have two children. Shay's blog and more information on her classes can be found at www.stefanosandshay.com.

TOMAS MONIZ is the founder and editor of (as well as writer for) the award-winning literary project *Rad Dad*. His book *Rad Families: A Celebration* will be released in 2016. He also wrote a novella, *Bellies and Buffalos,* a tender, chaotic road-trip story about friendship, family, and Flamin' Hot Cheetos. He is cofounder and cohost of the rambunctious monthly reading series Saturday Night Special. He's been making zines since the late Nineties. His most recent zines, *The Body is a Wild Wild Thing* and *addition / subtraction,* are available, but you have to write him a postcard: PO Box 3555, Berkeley, CA 94703.

Acknowledgments

MY ABSOLUTE GRATITUDE GOES out to everyone who helped me in making this book possible. First and foremost I'd like to thank my husband and partner, James Mogul, for his amazing support of my creative works and writing. Mr. Mogul, you are my rock, my family, my daddy, and your support means the world to me. I'd like to thank my child, Em, who is perhaps my greatest teacher in life and who has challenged me and inspired me in countless ways. Thank you for reminding me to stare at the clouds and splash in the puddles and to live in a world without time. Many thanks to Violet Blue, who first encouraged me to pitch and develop this book four years ago. Thank you for planting the seed. Thank you to my friends and fellow sexy mamas, as well as the Sexy Mamas Social Club. Your support and openness during my transition into motherhood and beyond provided a sense of strength and courage at a time when I needed it. Epic heaps of gratitude to my good friend Moorea Malatt for being such an inspiration in her own parenting and a wealth of knowledge, support, and amazing resources in the realm of raising a spirited feminist. You are a brilliant coach, teacher, and friend. I couldn't have written this book without the amazing assistance of my sitters, who do everything but sit—Freddie, Malic, Suzanne, Ellianna, and the amazing folks at the CCC after-school program. Thank you to my amazing assistant Gabriel Darling, who is a huge support in my creative life, and to Cara Kelsey, for helping me to create the time I needed to finish this book! Massive love and gratitude to all of our contributors who shared their stories and expertise in this book. Many thanks to Cleis Press for believing in this book, and to everyone who cheered me on through the process of writing it. You all inspire me so much. Thank you from the depths of my heart.

About the Author

MADISON YOUNG is an artist, author, certified sex educator, feminist pornographer, and mother. Young grew up in the suburban landscape of Southern Ohio before moving to San Francisco, California, in 2000. Young frequently teaches workshops and gives lectures on the topics of sexuality, feminist porn studies, motherhood and sexuality, and the politics of BDSM. She speaks around the world, including at academic institutions such as Yale University, Hampshire College, Northwestern University, the University of Toronto, the University of Minnesota, and the University of California, Berkeley. Young has been featured for her expertise in sex-positive culture in numerous documentaries and in television and media outlets such as Bravo, the Huffington Post, the *New York Times*, and HBO. Her writings have been published in books such as *The Ultimate Guide to Kink, Best Sex Writing 2013, Subversive Motherhood*, and *Coming Out Like a Porn Star*. Her memoir, *Daddy*, was published in February 2014 through Rare Bird/Barnacle Books, and her forthcoming book, *DIY Porn Handbook: Documenting Our Own Sexual Revolution*, will be out in August 2016 through Greenery Press. Madison Young lives in Berkeley, California, with her husband James and child Em.

photo by: Lydia Daniller.